Ventilators and Their Use

WHAT YOU WANT TO KNOW IF YOUR LOVED ONE IS ON LIFE SUPPORT

Ron Sanderson

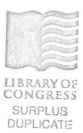

THE MAY PRESS

Honolulu, Hawai'i

Images of ventilators used with the permission of Hamilton Medical, Inc.

Ron Sanderson/The May Press

www.aboutventilators.com

Ventilators and Their Use/ Ron Sanderson. —1st ed.
ISBN 978-0-578-85671-1

To Lily, for she is the future; and to the myriad of ventilator patients and their loved ones.

Table of Contents

CHAPTER 1

Introduction to Ventilators and Their Use

In the spring of the year 2020 the word "ventilator" became a household word. This was because of the coronavirus pandemic that was causing thousands of additional people to need ventilators to try to survive the virus.

This book is about ventilators and the strange environment surrounding ventilators. Life support mechanical ventilators are complex medical devices that are typically used in the Intensive Care Unit (ICU). Mechanical ventilation is often initiated in the Emergency Room (ER).

People who have loved ones on ventilators have all sorts of questions and concerns about the well-being of their loved one. They have a strong desire to know what is going on in an environment that is nearly as foreign as the Space Station. The purpose of this book is to provide that information expediently and understandably; and in great depth for those who have the time and inclination to explore this astounding endeavor called artificial mechanical ventilation.

This book is organized as a quick, easy reference manual to address all questions that may come to the mind of family members and loved ones using ventilators. This first chapter contains a "Quick Reference", with simple clear bullet points addressing the issues in each chapter.

The following chapters explore this same topic in greater depth that will likely be challenging for the average person, but the intention is that it is understandable to anyone who is willing to dig in deeply. This book is primarily intended for lay people, although it may be of benefit to healthcare providers too.

The content in chapters 2 through 9 is arranged in order of what happens to people placed on a ventilator. Chapter 2, why do we use a ventilator in the first place? Chapter 3, what are ventilators? Chapter 4, who should be on a ventilator, or not? Chapter 5, how to put a person on a ventilator. Chapter 6, how to make changes to the ventilator while the patient is on it. Chapter 7, what are quality processes that protect ventilator patients? Chapter 8, how to discontinue or wean from the ventilator. Chapter 9, with all this knowledge we look at how specific diseases are typically managed on ventilators.

Regarding Chapter 6, if it seems too complex and difficult, please don't give up. Continue onto chapters 7, 8, and 9 which are less difficult to understand, and contain very important additional information.

This book is the author's best effort at sharing his knowledge, observations and opinions about ventilators and ventilator patient care; therefore, there are no references to medical journals. This is not a medical text. This is not a peer-reviewed scientific document. The information is meant to be true, science-based and to not include misinformation. The author is not trying to convince anyone of anything. Even though this book may sometimes seem like a technical manual, it is not. Do not go out and try to operate a ventilator after reading this book. Running a ventilator takes an ICU professional team and all the resources that implies. Finally, this book is for informational purposes only and is not a substitute for professional medical advice, diagnosis, or treatment.

This is not a book about ventilation of newborns and small children. There are many differences between mechanical ventilation of babies and larger people.

Having stated what the book is not, the author is a registered respiratory therapist and Doctor of Public Health. He has many years of experience in direct ventilator patient care in intensive care units. His knowledge of ventilator patients and families is front line. He has consulted with the largest ventilator manufacturers in the world as well as smaller ventilator companies in the development of new mechanical ventilators. In addition, he is a National and international speaker on the topic of mechanical ventilation at medical conferences.

Ventilators are called by other names like respirators, breathing machines, mechanical ventilators, or life support machines. Life support mechanical ventilators are not to be confused with air conditioners and fans for blowing air that are sometimes referred to as "ventilators". Ventilators are called "respirators", not to be confused with face mask devices that filter air or provide clean air in dusty or hazardous environments.

For clarity and simplicity, we will use the term ventilator.

Prior to the 2020 COVID-19 in the USA there were an estimated 10,000 people on ventilators daily. Every year we have 300,000 thousand people on ventilators. It needs to be borne in mind that in most acute care medical centers the average length of time a person spends on a ventilator is about 3 to 5 days. On one hand this average ventilator length of stay (LOS) is made smaller by a shorter length of ventilator stay of about one day or a few hours for many patients with healthy lungs who have had a successful major surgery and only spend a few hours or perhaps overnight on the ventilator. On the other hand, this average length of stay is increased and drawn-out to 3 - 5 days by most of the rest of the patients who spend five days to two weeks on ventilators for very serious medical/ surgical conditions. In addition to a very small number of people who need to remain on the ventilator for a period of several weeks to months. Usually after a person has been on a ventilator for more than one month they are considered a chronic ventilator patient which is not the primary subject of this book.

COVID-19 patients with Acute Respiratory Distress Syndrome (ARDS) are reported to spend 14 - 21 days on ventilators. This can be much longer or shorter depending on the specifics of each patient.

This information must not be misinterpreted, just because the average patient stays on the ventilator about 3 - 5 days does not mean that they come off the machine alive. There are two ways to come off the ventilator: 1) breathing spontaneously and alive or 2) not breathing and dead. The survival rate for ventilator patients can be very different from medical center to medical center and ICU to ICU depending on the types of patients admitted, criticality and type of the patients' diseases, the types of procedures performed, the amount of attention to end-of-life issues, the quality of medical care services provided, and policies regarding referral to more advanced institutions.

The overall estimated survival rate for a ventilator patient is 70 to 90%. For the sickest patients with Acute Respiratory Distress Syndrome (ARDS), it is 55 - 80% survival. COVID-19 patients often have ARDS. There are reports of 90% fatality among COVID-19 ventilator patients in New York City, Florida and China. In general, the sickest patients do the worst; the least complicated patients do much better. In some excellent intensive care units, the very sickest patients may have a better survival rate. At the same time some ventilator patients will not survive no matter where they are. They are just too sick and have too many body systems failing simultaneously to survive.

The opposite of survival rate is death rate or mortality rate. For ARDS the 25 to 45% mortality rate is worse than Russian roulette with a six-shooter, (approx. 16% chance of death). But this is more complicated than just the numbers. Just because a person survives their time on the ventilator does not say anything about their subsequent quality or quantity of life.

It is worth reminding ourselves that many ventilator patients have a healthful outcome, and go on to live many years of productive enjoyable life. Had they not been placed on a ventilator they would surely be dead.

Quick Reference for Chapter 1: Introduction

What are these machines?

Ventilators are very complex, electronic devices that control air and oxygen to blow breaths into a person to keep them alive. They are not all the same.

How do they work?

Simply put they are like a fireplace bellows, bicycle tire pump, or air mattress pump. But they are not simple, and usually don't contain pistons or bellows. There are a bunch of valves, connectors, tubes, and control knobs to regulate settings and alarms. The ventilator mixes oxygen and air and blows breaths into the patient.

When are ventilators used?

Anytime a person cannot breathe enough to stay alive. These are life support machines. They don't cure people. They just keep you alive until your underlying condition gets better, and you can breathe again by yourself.

Why would I want to be put on a ventilator?

Because you want to stay alive and think you have a chance of getting well if kept alive by the ventilator for a while.

When should I not go on a ventilator?

If your condition is terminal and you won't get well, it is probably better to die peacefully with family and friends with you, in palliative care.

How does it feel to be on a ventilator?

If a person is awake and has no pain killers, he/she feels terrible. Physically, you can't breathe, speak, eat, drink and you have to lie in bed. You can't get out to go to the bathroom, and must have a bedpan, bladder tube or diaper. You have to depend on others for everything. You may be in a lot of pain or have to take powerful medications. Mentally, you may be worrying about your loved ones, being a burden, or not being able to work or pay the bills.

Is it really that bad?

No, because the physician will provide the patient with pain killers and appropriate sedation to make the situation much more tolerable.

What is the chance of surviving being on a ventilator?

Survival depends on many factors most important of which is the reason the person was initially placed on the ventilator. Survival is usually higher than 50%. In many cases nearly 100%. With diseases like ARDS caused by COVID-19 the survival is sometimes as low as 10 - 40%.

How much do we have to pay for a patient on a ventilator?

If you have excellent insurance coverage, it could be free. If you don't have insurance, it costs a lot. ICU charges, physician fees, medicine, lab tests, ventilator charges and supplies may be between $20,000 and $40,000 per day.

If I don't have that kind of money, can the hospital refuse?

No, absolutely not. It is against the law, as well as against common decency. This should never happen.

If I cannot pay, what happens?

Whoever is responsible for the bill may go bankrupt, or if they don't have assets and the bill goes unpaid, the hospital loses money. Hopefully, the hospital won't go bankrupt. This is why everyone needs healthcare insurance. No one should have to go bankrupt or be hounded by bill collectors to save their life or their loved ones' lives.

Why does it cost so much?

Because you are mainly paying for the nurses, doctors and respiratory therapists who are running the ventilator, and expensive medicine, expensive tests and very expensive supplies.

If I am on a cheaper ventilator, do I pay less?

No, the pay is mainly for the health care workers, medicine, tests, and supplies to run the ventilator.

How much does the hospital make on a ventilator patient?

If the hospital gets the patient off the ventilator in a day or so, they might make a few thousand dollars. If the patient is on the ventilator longer than a week, it becomes very costly and the hospital is likely to lose money.

Who determines hospital charges and payments?

The hospital determines their charges, but don't get what they charge. Medicare and Medicaid determine what they will pay, and that is all the hospital gets. Other private insurance companies may pay more or less than Medicare and Medicaid depending on their coverage. Private people paying cash are expected to pay the whole bill but are usually given some discount if paid within a reasonable time.

How do ventilators affect people whose lives they save or prolong?

If the patient is on a ventilator for a short time and properly sedated, they may not remember anything and breathe just fine thereafter.

If the patient is super sick and on the ventilator for a long time, they can have PTSD and breathing problems for the rest of their life.

What about the families of these patients?

Families can visit the patients if the patient is not either highly infectious or immunocompromised. Meaning, if the patient can give the disease to others easily, or the patient is too weak to fight any germs the visitors bring in, visits may be denied. If the family is sick, they should stay out.

Who operates ventilators?

Respiratory therapists operate the ventilators according to physicians' specific orders. Nurses take care of the patient's overall problems and work with the respiratory therapists. Respiratory therapists should have a National Credential and a State License. This is the same with doctors and nurses.

Who are all the people working in the Intensive Care Unit (ICU)?

The ICU doctors are called intensivists, ICU nurses are amazingly competent and highly skilled nurses. Respiratory therapists operate the ventilator working closely with the intensivist and ICU nurse. There are also lab techs, x-ray techs, dietitians, specialist physicians, cleaning staff, pastors, nursing and healthcare students in the ICU.

Who do we ask questions and talk to about our loved one?

The team leader and the main source of information is a doctor. The other health care staff can answer questions related to their work. They should all have basically the same story.

How can I tell who is who in ICU?

The healthcare workers should all have visible ID badges and introduce themselves. It is ok to ask if it is hard to tell. It is a good idea to write down who you spoke to and what they said. It can get very confusing.

Why do some people say they don't want to be on life support or want "unplugged"?

Usually they are thinking that they are going to die and don't want to prolong the agony. Some people are misinformed and think everyone on a ventilator is brain dead. This is ignorant. When it comes down to dying of suffocation or going on a ventilator most people who have a decent chance to get well will choose the ventilator.

What if I really don't want to be on a breathing machine?

You need to have clear legal documents and instructions to your family, friends and the medical community to not save your life. It is a decision that is extremely difficult/almost impossible to make if you are already on the machine and the physician doesn't think you are going to die. You need to be very clear and have a POLST (Physician Orders for Life-Sustaining Treatment) and Advanced Directive. A POLST can be made by asking your primary physician and letting them know of your wishes. Advanced Directives is probably best made with advice of an attorney.

What if someone is brain dead and on a ventilator?

They can be taken off, only after it is clearly determined that their brain is dead. There are clear tests to determine brain death. More than one physician has to agree that the tests are correct before the ventilator is removed.

Quick Reference for Chapter 2: Why use a ventilator?

Why do we need to use a ventilator?

Any reason a person cannot breathe enough to stay alive. These are life support machines. They don't cure people. They just keep you alive until your underlying condition gets better, and you can breathe again by yourself.

Why would I want to be put on a ventilator?

Because you want to stay alive and think you have a chance of getting well if kept alive by the ventilator for a while.

How do we normally breathe?

Normally our diaphragm muscle contracts and sucks air in through our nose and mouth, the air down the windpipe into our lungs. This sucking is a pressure less than room pressure and is called negative pressure. Normal breathing is negative pressure respiration. Normally we breathe out by just relaxing our muscles.

How does the ventilator breathe people?

Ventilators blow air in through some kind of tube or sealed mask. A ventilator is like an air mattress pump, fireplace bellows, air compressor, or bicycle tire pump. They use positive pressure to blow the air into the person. Ventilators use positive pressure respiration. Ventilators do not breathe out; they just let the air come out passively like normal breathing.

Why does the physician sometimes use "medical coma"?

"Medical coma" is the use of sedatives and perhaps paralytic drugs to make the ventilator patient relax and not resist the machine. "Medical Coma" has the advantage of being reversible in a few hours when the medical team decides it is best for the patient.

More specifically, why do people need a ventilator?

People need a life support ventilator for one or more of the following reasons:

Overall reason: The patient cannot move enough air in and out of their lungs by themselves.

General reasons:

1. They cannot get enough oxygen from their lungs into their blood.
2. Their normal breathing tubes (bronchial tubes) are obstructed, too narrow or blocked.
3. Their lungs or chest wall are too stiff, leathery or fibrous.
4. Their central stimulus to breathe from the brain is impaired or absent.
5. Their breathing muscles are too weak to get enough breath.
6. Their blood going to their lungs is not matching with the air being breathed in.

The doctor may know in advance that this person will have respiratory failure. There are many specific diseases and causes of these general problems, but it all comes down to these six conditions or circumstances.

ARDS from COVID-19 seems to be reason #1. Often the doctor can predict this oxygenation failure in a COVID-19 patient and place them on a ventilator before the patient becomes too stressed, reason #7. It is beginning to appear that COVID-19 also causes reason #6.

What is a normal sized breath and respiratory rate?
Normally people breathe in somewhere between a cup and a pint of air (200 - 500ml.) each breath. We normally breathe 10 - 15 times per minute.

How big a breath can a person take when breathing in and out as deeply as possible?
3 - 5 quarts (3 - 5 liters) and this is quite different between normal people depending on age, sex, and height.

What causes us to breathe without thinking about it all the time?
The unconscious brain signals the breathing muscles to work all the time. The brain is monitoring the carbon dioxide and oxygen levels in the blood, as well as some other signals from the body.

Quick Reference for Chapter 3: The Ventilator

How do ventilators breathe for people?

They push air into the patient's lungs from a high-pressure gas source or some sort of piston-like device. This positive pressure is the opposite of normal breathing where we suck air into our lungs using primarily the diaphragm muscle. Sucking and vacuum create negative pressure. Ventilators create positive pressure, the opposite of normal breathing.

How is the ventilator connected to the patient?

A tube called an endotracheal tube is inserted through the patient's nose or mouth down into the windpipe where a balloon on the end of the tube is sealed. The ventilator is connected to the other end of the tube near the lips or nose.

A non-invasive mask that is sealed to the patient's face covering the nose and mouth is usually a short-term connection. The ventilator is connected to the mask.

A tracheostomy tube is a surgically placed tube through the front of the neck directly into the windpipe just below the Adam's Apple. Tracheostomy tubes have a balloon on the end to seal the airway. The ventilator is connected to the tracheostomy tube on an adapter sticking out below the patient's chin. This tube allows the patient to be able to talk, eat and drink even though it is difficult.

What happens if the power goes off?

The ventilator is powered by electricity. If the power goes off or someone accidentally unplugs the ventilator it will alarm like crazy. Most ventilators contain a back-up battery that immediately takes over and keep it going for 30 mins to a few hours. In addition, if the electric company has a power failure, the medical center has a back-up diesel electric generator. The back-up generator is tested monthly and supplies electricity to special red colored electrical outlets. The ventilator should always be connected to a red electrical outlet.

What happens if the oxygen to the ventilator gets unplugged?
Again, it will alarm and staff will need to plug it back in right away or connect the ventilator to a portable oxygen tank.

How often do ventilators malfunction?
Almost never. In the event of failure of any of the important systems there are alarms and safety mechanisms in place to ensure the patient's safety.

How are ventilators cleaned between patients?
The entire outside of the machine is wiped with disinfectant and all the parts in contact with the patients are single patient use and thrown away, or re-used, after sterilization in surgical sterilizers. The machines are sampled periodically by infection control staff to check for cleanliness.

When is the ventilator checked for proper function?
It is checked and documented by the respiratory therapist every 2 - 4 hours while on the patient. Between patient's use the ventilator undergoes complete and serious checking of every important function and alarm systems.

How much does it cost to buy a ventilator?

Commonly $5,000 to $50,000 and like most things you get more features as the price increases. Prices vary between different countries.

How long does a ventilator last?

Lifespan of a ventilator is considered to be 10 years. Well-engineered ventilators can last longer with good maintenance and good treatment.

How are the ICU staff able to transport a ventilator patient to surgery or special procedures?

The ventilator is connected to a portable oxygen tank and allowed to run on battery power. In addition, the nurse has a portable monitor and IV pumps that go along with the patient.

You may see ICU staff hand ventilating the patient with a manual resuscitation bag and oxygen tank during transport. This should not be done except in a dire emergency. The National standard of practice is to transport ventilator patients on their ventilator or a special transport mechanical ventilator. The manual resuscitator cannot match the ventilator volumes, oxygen level and respiratory rate and is dangerous to the patient.

What information is on the display screen on the front of the ventilator?

This screen displays ventilator settings, an amazing amount of information from patient, alarm settings, and may connect to the patient's electronic medical record and the ICU main nursing station monitor.

What is a pulse oximeter?

A pulse oximeter sensor commonly clips to the patient's fingertip like a clothespin, only more gently, and shines light through the finger checking light absorbed by the pulsing arterial blood. If the patient has low blood pressure or cold hands, the pulse oximeter may not be accurate. The pulse oximeter has other sensors that may clip to the ear or stick to the forehead. All of these probes must be used as designed to be accurate. No finger probes should be clipped to other body parts. If you ask the ICU staff why the finger probe is being used on the ear, you may hear them say that they are getting a "good reading"; unfortunately, that is a false reading and they just happen to like it.

What is a capnograph or end-tidal carbon dioxide detector?

The capnograph sensor is usually placed in the ventilator hoses going to and from the patient. It allows the ICU staff to measure carbon dioxide without taking a blood sample. Carbon dioxide level is the measurement of effectiveness of ventilation. This type of carbon dioxide detector is non-invasive, doesn't poke holes in the patient, reads out constantly, and is reasonably accurate when interpreted correctly. It does need to be checked against arterial blood gas samples occasionally.

Quick Reference for Chapter 4: Assessment of Breathing and Indications for Mechanical Ventilation

What if I don't want to go on a ventilator?

You can refuse any medical treatment, even against professional advice. A big problem is that a person is so sick or unconscious at the time a ventilator is needed. If a person doesn't want to go on a ventilator it is very important to plan ahead.

How do I plan ahead to refuse to be on a ventilator?

You should make a POLST (Physician Orders for Life-Sustaining Treatment). A POLST is an abbreviated type of Advanced Directive that states directly "Do or Do not Resuscitate" if the patient has no pulse or is not breathing. The POLST should be made with your doctor.

The POLST needs to be signed and made readily available to Emergency Medical Services (Ambulance or Emergency Room) personnel.

What are Advanced Directives?

The patient may want to have "advanced directives" to clearly direct their end-of-life care. These are legal documents like Power of Attorney or Last Will and Testament. Most medical centers will assist patients to execute such documents.

How did the doctor decide to put my loved one on a ventilator?

The doctor will only place patients on a ventilator if they cannot breathe, if there is no less invasive solution to the problem, or if the patient will soon lose the ability to breathe.

What is BiPAP or non-invasive ventilation (NIV)?

"BiPAP' is a proprietary name commonly misused to refer to non-invasive ventilation (NIV). It is like using Kleenex for facial tissue or Xerox for a photocopy. NIV is hooking a ventilator up to the patient with a face mask. It is called non-invasive because a tube is not inserted down the patient's throat. NIV can be very effective over the short term, but most practitioners are reluctant to use it for many days. In addition, if high levels of PEEP are necessary the face mask may leak too much.

Quick Reference for Chapter 5: Initiating Mechanical Ventilation

What is "tidal volume"?

The size of one single breath is called tidal volume. It is usually about one cup to one pint of air 200-500 ml. The tidal volume is a setting on the ventilator so each patient can get the right sized breath. When the ventilator gives a breath, it is called a "machine breath". When the patient takes their own breath, it is called a spontaneous breath. Both machine breaths or spontaneous breaths have some set or measured tidal volume.

What is a reasonable percentage of oxygen?

If the patient does not have an oxygenation problem the ventilator is usually set to give 30 - 40% oxygen. If in an emergency no one knows the patient's oxygen level or problem, the ventilator is started at 100% oxygen, the maximum amount.

What is PEEP?

PEEP is Positive End-Expiratory Pressure. This means at the end of a breath out, the ventilator holds some pressure against the airway and the lungs to "hold them open" between the breaths. It is believed that the endotracheal tubes may allow the lungs to exhale deeper and become more flat than usual. So, 5 - 10 mmHg of PEEP is most always used. PEEP is also used to help keep the lungs open in ARDS. It is like blowing up a balloon. It is very hard at first then becomes easy. If you were going to let a balloon deflate and blow it up again, it would make sense to not let it go clear flat, so it is easier to reinflate.

What is a "medical coma"?

Medical coma is a term used to describe the use of sedative drugs used for putting a person to "sleep". There are also pain killer drugs like Morphine (opiates) that affect a patient's consciousness. In addition, there are "paralytic" drugs to keep patients from moving too much or at all. Ventilator patients in a medical coma are probably on more than one of the drugs above for their own benefit.

What is a "mode of ventilation"?

Most simply it is the way the ventilator breathes the patient or allows them to help in the breathing. Control mode is the ventilator doing all the breathing using the breaths set by the respiratory therapist. Spontaneous mode is the ventilator allowing the patient to take a breath whenever they want and take the size of breath they want. In fact, there are many ventilator modes that combine both control and spontaneous breathing. In the end, mode of ventilation is not simple at all.

What is "pressure support"?

If a patient on the ventilator is in a mode of ventilation that allows spontaneous breaths, pressure support is a little breath of air given by the ventilator to boost what the patient was able to do on their own. With little or no pressure support the patient is doing all the work to breathe. With a lot of pressure support all the patient might have to do is just barely start to take a breath and then do nothing.

How do they know the ventilator is set correctly when it is first attached?

Fortunately, the doctors know what a patient will need, so they take their best guess and hook the patient up watching closely and looking at the monitors. If the patient looks about right, they will draw an arterial blood gas to check after about 30 mins.

Quick Reference for Chapter 6: Optimizing Mechanical Ventilation

Why do they keep changing settings on the ventilator?

The patient's respiratory condition often changes, so the ventilator has to be changed to best match the patient's situation.

What is the most important ventilator setting to ask about?

Ask, "What is the percentage of oxygen the patient is on and how much PEEP?" Hopefully oxygen is 40% or less and PEEP is 10 cmH$_2$O or less. If oxygen percentage and PEEP are getting higher the patient is getting worse. If the oxygen percentage and PEEP are getting lower the patient is improving.

Ask, "Is the patient breathing at all, if so how much?"
x
Generally, it is good for patients to be awake and doing some breathing or assisting the ventilator. If they are not awake or breathing ask, "Why?" There are many reasons why that are good to hear about from the intensivist or ICU staff.

What is an artery and a vein?

Arteries are blood vessels that take fresh oxygenated blood out to all parts of the body. When we feel a pulse, we are feeling an artery pumping
Veins are blood vessels that bring back blood that has been used by the body to the heart to get pumped to the lungs and refreshed. Most blood test samples are taken from veins.

What are arterial blood gases or "blood gases"?

A lab test to check how much oxygen and carbon dioxide are in the blood. This is the best test result to check the patient's breathing and use of the ventilator.

Why are blood gases taken from arteries instead of veins like most blood samples?

Blood in the arteries has just come from the lungs, so if we want to see how the lungs are working, ventilating and oxygenating, it's the best place to look.

What is a normal oxygen level in the blood?

P_aO_2 = 80 - 100 cmH_2O. when breathing regular air, room air. P_aO_2 is a unit of measuring an amount (partial pressure) of oxygen (O_2) in "a" (arterial blood). "cmH_2O" is a unit of pressure. What is most important is that this is different than pulse oximeter readings and more accurate.

What are considered high and low oxygen levels?

A "High P_aO_2" is more than 100 cmH_2O. High oxygen is not a problem. High oxygen is just unnecessary and not particularly helpful. Low oxygen starts at 50 to 70 cmH_2O or lower and is usually corrected by increasing the percentage of oxygen the patient is given or increasing PEEP (Positive End Expiratory Pressure). PEEP is a pressure the ventilator holds in the lungs to help with oxygenation.

Can people survive with seriously low oxygen levels, less than 40 cmH₂O?

Seriously low oxygen is not tolerable. The heart and brain suffer very quickly, and the person will begin to die.

Why does the red blood cell count (hemoglobin and hematocrit) matter?

Oxygen is carried from the lungs to the rest of the body on hemoglobin in red blood cells. You can think of them as little buckets full of oxygen. If there aren't enough red blood cells, the body tissues, particularly the heart and brain, don't get enough oxygen.

What is normal hemoglobin and hematocrit?

Hemoglobin equals 12 to 15 grams per deciliter, hematocrit is 36 to 45%. Hemoglobin is a molecule in the blood that carries most of the oxygen. It is important that it is above 8 or 9 gm/dl or the blood is not able to carry enough oxygen from the lungs to the patient's body.

What is a normal carbon dioxide, P_aCO_2, level in the arterial blood?

P_aCO_2 = 35 - 45 cmH₂O when breathing enough to get carbon dioxide (bad air) out of the body. P_aCO_2 is a unit of measuring an amount (partial pressure) of carbon dioxide (CO_2) in "a" (arterial blood). "cmH₂O" is a unit of pressure.

What are considered high and low carbon dioxide levels?

Carbon dioxide, P_aCO_2, over 50 or 60 is usually corrected by increasing the respiratory rate of the ventilator. Carbon dioxide less than 25 to 30 is usually corrected by decreasing the respiratory rate of the ventilator. High and low carbon dioxide also affect the acid-alkaline balance of the blood and body.

What else do blood gases measure?

They measure the acid or alkaline level of the blood, called pH. Our blood is usually neutral with a pH = 7.40 (7.35 - 7.45). If the blood gets acidic or basic it goofs up all kinds of chemical reactions in the body and must be corrected.

If the patient is breathing better, what is changed first?

Let's say we have now allowed time for the patient/ventilator relationship to equilibrate and have received results of our first assessment of this situation. Alternatively, we could say that the patient/ventilator relationship is constantly changing, and we are at any point of maintaining the patient on artificial ventilation. Here the healthcare team will try to support the patient's breathing with the greatest amount of comfort, least amount of interference and least number of complications. More specifically, the least amount of pressure, volume, mechanical breaths, and oxygen necessary to support the patient without overtaxing the patient's condition will be used. This may mean that the ventilator does all the breathing at high pressures and high oxygen percentage, say 60 -100% or it may mean that the ventilator supplies minimal pressure support to a spontaneous breathing patient on a low oxygen percentage, say 30%

The physician will direct the changing of mode of ventilation, tidal volume, respiratory rate, F_1O_2 and PEEP either by direct order or via pre-approved protocol. Other ventilator settings or adjustments fine tuning the patient/ventilator will be changed by the respiratory therapist. All changes will be documented in the patient's record.

Review: Why do patients need a ventilator

- Their lungs or chest wall are too stiff, leathery or fibrous.
- Their breathing tubes (bronchial tubes) are obstructed, too narrow or blocked.
- The breathing muscles are not getting a signal from the brain to breathe.
- Their breathing muscles are too weak to get enough breath.
- Their blood going to their lungs is not matching with the air being breathed in.
- They cannot get enough oxygen from their lungs into their blood.

The doctor may know in advance that this person will have respiratory failure. Then they are put on a ventilator before they experience respiratory failure.

These reduce down to basically two problems:

Ventilatory failure – primary assessment is P_aCO_2 – adjust by changing respiratory rate
Oxygenation failure – primary assessment is P_aO_2 – adjust by changing oxygen percentage or PEEP

COVID-19 as we understand it is primarily reason #6 and possibly #5 causing the development of Acute Respiratory Distress Syndrome (ARDS). This will be followed by problem #1. We hope the physician can see this coming before the patient goes into respiratory and cardiac arrest (stops breathing and no heartbeat).

Quick Reference for Chapter 7: Protocols and Best Practices

Why is the head of the bed up all the time?

This is to prevent fluid from the stomach, secretions from the nose and mouth going back down and leak into the lungs. When this happens, it can cause pneumonia. We want to prevent ventilator associated pneumonia.

Why does the patient have inflating balloon-like cuffs around their lower legs?

These are to prevent the formation of blood clots in the legs. If a blood clot breaks loose from a vein in the leg it will end up in the patient's heart or lungs. When people lie in bed for a long time this is much more likely.

What is a Spontaneous Breathing Trial (SBT)?

An SBT is the ICU staff giving ventilator patients a chance to breathe on their own each morning. This is done after most sedation wears off. If the patient can successfully breathe for 30 mins to 2 hours. It may be time to get rid of the ventilator.

What if the patient does not pass the SBT?

That happens as often as not. The patient will be safely returned to ventilator support, and the ICU staff will try again tomorrow if appropriate.

Quick Reference for Chapter 8: Weaning Patient off Mechanical Ventilation

How long must a patient be on a ventilator?

The patient must be on the ventilator until the underlying causes of their respiratory failure have been resolved or reversed. The least amount of time on a ventilator is always best as being on a ventilator is a dangerous situation for the patient. At the same time the ICU staff try to avoid taking the patient off the ventilator too soon and then have the patient "crash," requiring them to put the patient back on the ventilator.

How does the doctor know the ventilator can be taken off the patient?

In the simplest cases the patient wakes up from anesthesia or a temporary condition is reversed quickly, and the doctor knows the patient will be fine off the ventilator.

In most other cases the intensivist orders a number of tests of the patient's ability to breathe and cough, asks the respiratory therapist and ICU nurse, and does an SBT. If the patient is successful with SBT for 30 mins. to 2 hours, probably they can come off the ventilator.

Quick Reference for Chapter 9: Ventilator Use with Specific Diseases

What can we expect if our loved one is on a ventilator? Because:

Post-op Cardiac Surgery - The patient is usually off the ventilator in a few hours to overnight. If it is longer than that their condition is complex.

Other Major Surgery - there are many different major surgeries that land a person on a ventilator. Occasionally they just need to wake up and have the ventilator removed. In other cases, they may need to be on one for a few days.

Bronchial Asthma - ventilators are the life saving device for people with near-fatal asthma attacks. If the severe asthma symptoms can be reversed, the patient often comes off in one day. If the severe asthma symptoms cannot be broken, the patient may be on the ventilator a few days.

Overdose, sedatives - If this patient did not suck stomach contents down in their lungs when they passed out, they should be off the ventilator in a few hours to overnight. If they aspirated stomach contents, likely they will develop ARDS, see below.

Acute Respiratory Distress Syndrome (ARDS) - If your loved one has ARDS, they will likely be on the ventilator for 1 - 4 weeks. The chance of their dying on the ventilator is quite possible, so hope for the best, but have realistic expectations.

Heart Attack - Once the heart problem is under control the patient can usually come off the ventilator. Some heart attacks are definitely worse than others and the patient can have other major organ damage (brain, lungs, kidneys, etc.). These patients will most likely be on the ventilator longer.

Obesity - These patients might be on the ventilator for weeks or months until their weight can be reduced. If this happens, they might get a tracheostomy tube and only be able to talk, eat and speak with difficulty. Be sure to cooperate with the ICU staff and do not bring in food for the patient.

Brain trauma and brain surgery - These patients have a wide variety of reasons for the need to be on the ventilator. It is important to speak to the neurosurgeon, neurologist and intensivist to understand the need for the ventilator.

Neuromuscular disease - These patients may be having a short disruption of their medication or a relatively reversible problem with their underlying disease and be off the ventilator soon. In many cases the neuromuscular disease is progressively getting worse and they will possibly be on the ventilator for the rest of their life.

Trauma/Injury - These patients have a wide variety of reasons to need the ventilator. It is important to speak to the surgeon, and intensivist to understand the need for the ventilator.

Near-Drowning - Near drowning patients mostly do not need hospital care. Those who get their lungs full of water will go on a ventilator, and most will have ARDS. Again, the survival from ARDS is 20 - 40%.

Chronic Obstructive Pulmonary Disease

COPD combines two similar diseases, pulmonary emphysema and chronic bronchitis. COPD obstructs the bronchial tubes and alveoli (air sacs) by the tissue becoming fibrotic.

 We try to avoid placing COPD patients on ventilators because there is little or no ability to reverse the underlying condition and they will be "stuck" on the ventilator. It is very important for advanced COPD patients to have end of life conversations with their physicians, so everyone knows what the patient wants (see Chapter 1, advanced directives and POLST)

Acute exacerbation of COPD can be caused by pneumonia. In this case the underlying cause can be reversed, and the ventilator discontinued after a few days.

Each time this happens the patient ends up a little worse off and by the third intubation it is most likely the patient will become a chronic ventilator patient. Few people want to live like that; however, some people might choose to stay on a ventilator.

Pneumonia (bacterial, viral, fungal)

Pneumonia infections from bacteria, virus or other germs can be acquired at home or in the hospital. It may first seem like a common cold or flu, and then the patient starts having severe problems breathing. COVID-19 is a viral pneumonia. Pneumonia often develops into ARDS. The goal is to reverse the infection. This is easier with bacteria that may be killed by antibiotics. Unfortunately, viruses are not killed by antibiotics and there are few medicines effective against fungal infections. In these cases, we have to give the patients medicines that can help their immune system fight the infections and keep the patient alive in the meantime. The outcome for ventilator patients with pneumonia are much better if ARDS does not develop. If it does develop into ARDS the outcome is less than 70% survival like ARDS.

CHAPTER 2

Why Ventilators?

People need a life support ventilator for one or more of the following reasons:

Overall reason: The patient cannot breathe enough air in and out of their lungs by themselves.

Main reasons:

1. Their normal breathing tubes (bronchial tubes) are obstructed, too narrow or blocked.
2. Their lungs or chest wall are too stiff, leathery or fibrous.
3. Their central stimulus to breathe from the brain is impaired or absent.
4. Their breathing muscles are too weak to get enough breath.
5. They cannot get enough oxygen through their lungs into their blood.
6. Blood going to their lungs for oxygen is blocked from getting to lung areas with air.
7. The doctor knows in advance that this person will have respiratory failure.

There are many causes of these main problems, but it all comes down to these seven conditions or circumstances.

ARDS from COVID-19 seems to be reason #5. Often the doctor can predict this oxygenation failure and place them on a ventilator before the patient becomes too stressed, reason #7. It also seems COVID-19 causes #6.

The remainder of this chapter explores these situations in detail starting with normal breathing. The normal breathing section includes respiratory anatomy, exploring the parts of the respiratory system and physiology looking at how our breathing works. This will be a good reference to many instances later in the book. These in-depth sections are followed by how the respiratory system can fail with explanation of the two general categories of respiratory failure that are oxygenation failure and ventilation failure.

Normal breathing

Human beings have been breathing for a very long time. Depending on whether you believe in creation or evolution, it is for thousands or millions of years. We do an excellent job of breathing; so, perhaps, it would be wise to briefly explore normal breathing in order to best understand why we would choose to artificially take over this function with a mechanical ventilator.

"In goes the good air; out goes the bad air," the purpose of breathing is to bring oxygen (O_2) into the lungs where it diffuses across the alveolocapillary membranes into the blood. This happens deep in the lungs on a microscopic level. Then, from the lungs, oxygenated blood goes back to the heart and gets pumped through the arteries to the tissue cells all over the body. This ultimately provides oxygen for the chemical "fires" of oxidation (burning) of sugar inside our cells. Cellular respiration produces energy, carbon dioxide, and water. That energy is used to power all of our bodily functions. The carbon dioxide exits cells to the blood and gets pumped by the heart through the veins back to the lungs where it diffuses out of the blood into the lungs and is ventilated to the atmosphere by breathing. "In goes the good air; out goes bad air" simplistically is an accurate statement. We need to remember that the process of cellular respiration requires two pumps. Lungs are a bellows pumping air, moving oxygen into, and CO_2 out of, the lungs. The heart interfaces with the lungs and pumps oxygenated blood from the lungs to all body cells and returns blood with low oxygen and increased CO_2 to the lungs. The first pump is an air pump, ventilation. The second pump is a liquid pump, circulation.

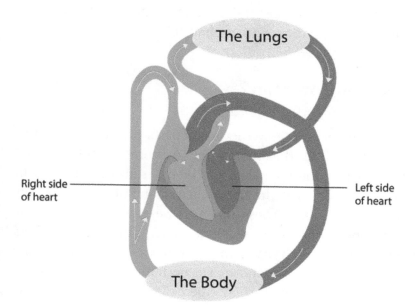

Breathing refers to our normal taking air into and expelling air from our lungs. Ventilation in this context is the supply of air in and out of the lungs; especially by artificial means; ventilators. Respiration is the process of burning sugar with oxygen and producing carbon dioxide in the cells. This is also referred to as "cellular respiration" for clarity. At one time people used the terms "internal respiration" for cellular respiration and "external respiration" for ventilation.

This is why ventilators are also called "breathing machines" or "respirators". However, they most definitely are mechanical ventilators, ventilating air in and out of the lungs. Again, not to be confused with room fans or building air conditioners moving air in and out of buildings.

To further muddy the definition, medical professionals determine the breathing rate as "counting respirations"; so many "breaths per minute" and it is documented as "frequency"; frequency of respiration, with a small "f".

Normal Lung Anatomy

The diagrams below show the major parts of the airways and the lung as well as the microscopic anatomy of the air sacs (alveoli), where the air meets the blood from the heart. It is important to note that the upper airways humidify and warm air entering the body. These upper airways are bypassed with artificial tubes when we use ventilators. Also note the area called the pharynx. The pharynx is the back of the mouth or throat. The pharynx is a problematic area as both the lungs through the larynx and the stomach through the esophagus divide here on the way down and merge here on the way up. Likewise, the nose and mouth merge here on the way in and divide here on the way out. Somehow, we manage to breathe air from our nose or mouth through this intersection, and it goes in the larynx, not the esophagus. Somehow, we manage to eat and drink with the food and water going through this intersection, and it goes in the esophagus, not in the lungs. If food and water, go into the larynx it causes coughing and choking to get it out before going down in the lungs. If air goes down the esophagus, we burp it out. The common artificial airway used with ventilators, the endotracheal tube, has to be put through the nose or mouth and around the corner to go into the larynx.

Upper Airways

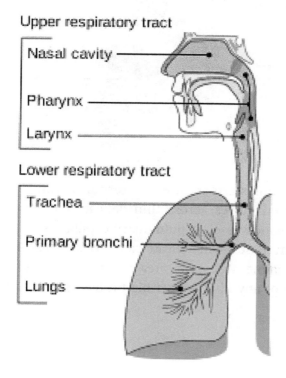

We have two lungs one on the left of the heart and one on the right. The right lung has three lobes and the left lung has two. The trachea splits to a right and left main bronchus for each lung. These bronchi branch 20 to 23 times before they become air sacs or alveoli where exchange of oxygen and carbon dioxide occurs with the blood.

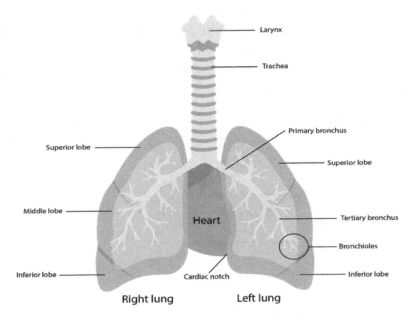

The alveolocapillary unit starts at the end or terminal bronchiole. This is where oxygen moves across thin delicate membranes into the tiny lung blood vessel or pulmonary capillaries, where carbon dioxide from these small delicate capillaries diffuse back into the lung for exhaling. When this area gets attacked by virus, bacteria, or trauma of any kind we get big problems being able to breathe.

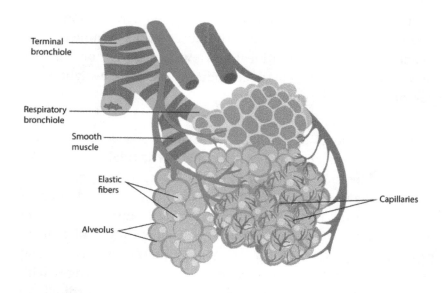

Terminal bronchiole
Respiratory bronchiole
Smooth muscle
Elastic fibers
Alveolus
Capillaries

Breathing Rate, Tidal Volume, and Minute Volume

Normally without any conscious effort we breathe 12 to 20 times per minute while resting. During this minute we typically move a total of about 5 L of air. (1 liter = 0.95 quarts) in and out of our lungs. 16 breaths or 5 liters times 1440 minutes in a day equals about 23000 breaths or 7200 L. (1900 gallons) of ventilation per day. That's quite a bit of work to do without even giving it a thought. The abbreviation for respiratory rate is "f", for frequency of breaths per minute.

Tidal volume (TV) is the volume of a normal single breath, about 300 to 500 ml, less than one pint. Tidal volume varies among individuals according to the person's height, age and gender.

Shorter people, older people, and women have respectively smaller tidal volumes. A rule of thumb says tidal volume is equal to about 3 ml per pound ideal body weight (IBW) or 7 ml/Kg IBW. Ideal body weight is considered the ideal weight for a person, not too skinny, not too fat.

Minute volume (VE) is the total volume of gas entering (or leaving) the lung per minute. It is equal to the tidal volume (TV) multiplied by the respiratory rate (f). Minute volume = VE = TV x f. At rest, a normal person moves ~400 ml/breath x 10 breath/ min = 4000 ml/min. Minute volume is an important concept because our minute volume needs to match our metabolic rate to provide enough oxygen to keep up with cellular respiration and get rid of excess carbon dioxide. Metabolic rate changes with exercise or fever, so minute volume must adjust accordingly to keep enough oxygen available. If a person is on a ventilator, we have to do this for them.

Vital Capacity and Functional Residual Capacity

Vital capacity is another measure of breathing volume. It is much larger than tidal volume. Inspiratory vital capacity is how big a breath a person can take in from the point of deepest exhalation to deepest inhalation. Expiratory vital capacity is how big a breath a person can blow out from the point of deepest inhalation to deepest exhalation. They should be about the same. Normal vital capacity is about 3 - 5 liters varying according to height, age, and gender.

The diagram below shows tidal volume, vital capacity and a couple of other lung volumes and capacities that are used when discussing mechanical ventilators. This tracing is made in a pulmonary function laboratory. You can see the person being tested is first taking three normal relaxed breaths, tidal volume. Then they breathe in as deeply as possible making the line go up to a maximum level. Then they blow that deep breath all the way out as deeply as possible. The line on the tracing goes down as far as possible for the patient and then they take one normal breath back in.

You will note that Functional Residual Capacity (FRC) is the amount of air left in the lungs after a normal exhalation. Look under the first three breaths in the spirogram below. At the end of resting exhalation there is quite a large volume of remaining in the lung, FRC. FRC keeps our lungs from going completely flat between breaths and is a reservoir or gas tank to keep carbon dioxide from going to zero each breath. If our lungs went empty or flat at the end of each breath it would be a big problem. Imagine blowing up a balloon. It is very hard at first and then when partially inflated the balloon is much easier to blow up as it gets bigger. Likewise, if our lungs went completely flat between breaths, it would probably be too much effort to keep breathing very long. To make better sense of this, please identify tidal volume, vital capacity and functional residual capacity in the diagram below.

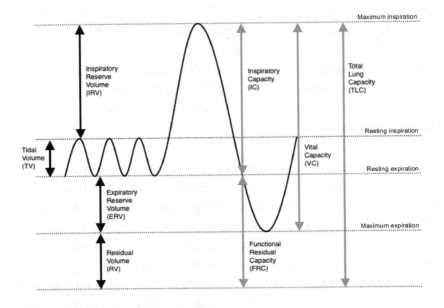

Exercise and Other Breathing Maneuvers

Exercise may increase ventilation of the lungs to greater than 100 breaths per minute and a minute volume of 100 L. Our bodies have an impressive respiratory reserve. Maximum Voluntary Ventilation is the name of a 15 sec. maximum effort pulmonary function test where people breathe as fast and deeply as possible. Normal people can produce a maximal voluntary ventilation of 120 - 170 L/min., depending on height, gender and age. Keep in mind we can only breathe at our maximum voluntary ventilation for a short time; even 12 to 20 seconds is uncomfortable. World-class marathon runners maintain a minute volume of around 100 liters per minute while running. That is 20 times normal for more than 2 hours.

Normal quiet breathing is unconscious; however, we can consciously perform many respiratory maneuvers, for example, talking, singing, whistling, horn playing, coughing, throat clearing, sneezing, spitting, breath-holding, pill-taking, and many more. So, what keeps us breathing?

Respiratory Regulation

There are several mechanisms of the automatic control of human breathing. There are respiratory centers in the brainstem that receive information from receptors in blood vessels, reflexes from the lungs, messages from the conscious mind, as well as detectors in the brainstem itself.

Breath to breath we breathe as a result of constant stimulation from carbon dioxide in arterial blood. We breathe to keep our arterial carbon dioxide level between 35 to 45 mmHg. The arterial CO_2 level between 35 to 45 is important to know. If a person who is maintained on a ventilator is outside this range, there should be a reasonable medical explanation. The brain keeps our quiet breathing hardly noticeable by responding to CO_2 stimulation in addition to these reflexes from the lungs and other rhythm centers in the brain stem. Please see the diagram on the next page.

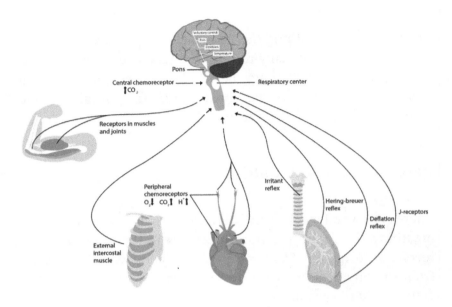

It is important to mention here that if the oxygen level in arterial blood gets quite low and our blood gets acidotic (low pH) these factors will stimulate respirations and override the normal CO_2 drive to breathe. There are a few situations where hypoxia (low oxygen) and acidosis help explain what is going on with a ventilator patient. Please see the section on COPD patient on ventilators, Chapter 9, for further explanation.

The explanations above are quite simplistic; however, they represent the better-known regulatory processes of breathing.

Mechanics of Normal Ventilation (not mechanical ventilation)

This is a terribly exciting topic; because, most of us haven't thought about it much, and the idea that a container (our chest) can get larger when the walls of the container contract around it seems very unusual and not what we would normally think is possible. The lungs are encased in a fairly rigid, bony, muscular cage. The ribs are covered with, and bounded by, muscles. The thoracic cage is made up of the ribs held together in the back by the spine and the front by the sternum or breastbone.

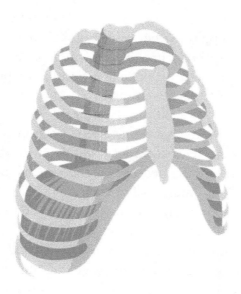

Illustration of the chest cage with the diaphragm muscle being the bottom of the cage.

Thoracic cavity is shaped like an inverted cone and has a muscle called the diaphragm as the bottom wall. The diaphragm does about 80% of normal breathing work and the intercostal muscles between each rib does about 20% of normal breathing. For those who eat meat intercostal muscles from pigs and cows make delicious barbeque.

When the muscles contract it causes the chest to expand, increasing its volume and decreasing the pressure inside the lungs to below atmospheric (slight vacuum). This slight subatmospheric pressure difference, approximately -2 centimeters of water (cmH$_2$0), causes air to flow in through our nose or mouth into our lungs, we breathe in. When the muscles relax the cage collapses creating a slight positive pressure (+ 2 cmH$_2$0) and the air flows out; we breathe out. This slight vacuum breathing in is called negative pressure breathing because it is slightly lower than air pressure outside our body in the atmosphere or air around us. Normal breathing is negative pressure. Ventilators push air into our lungs and is called positive pressure.

Let's think of the thoracic cage, as a box with muscles on the outside when the muscles contract it would seem that the box would collapse. However, because of the special arrangement of our diaphragm and muscles between the ribs (intercostals), just the opposite occurs. The chest expands when these muscles contract. When the muscles of the diaphragm contract, the diaphragm descends into the abdominal cavity and contraction of the intercostals cause the ribs to move out and up. The chest volume expands. Therefore, normal inhalation or inspiration is an active process. Exhalation is just passive relaxation of these same muscles. A patient receiving mechanical ventilation also has relatively normal passive exhalation. The mechanical ventilator only pushes the breath in.

The illustration below shows the many muscles involved in breathing. Please note there are primary muscles used during relaxed and deep breathing, and there are accessory muscles used during deep breaths in or out.

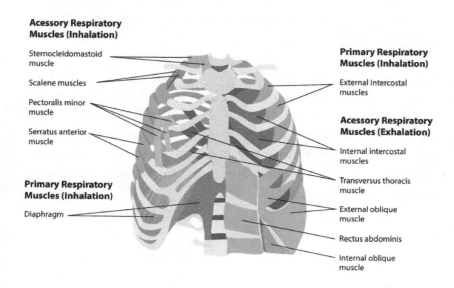

Acessory Respiratory Muscles (Inhalation)

Sternocleidomastoid muscle

Scalene muscles

Pectoralis minor muscle

Serratus anterior muscle

Primary Respiratory Muscles (Inhalation)

Diaphragm

Primary Respiratory Muscles (Inhalation)

External Intercostal muscles

Acessory Respiratory Muscles (Exhalation)

Internal intercostal muscles

Transversus thoracis muscle

External oblique muscle

Rectus abdominis

Internal oblique muscle

The primary muscles of ventilation are the diaphragm and the intercostal muscles. The diaphragm does 80% of the work of normal breathing and the intercostals 20%. This can become a very important issue if during heart surgery or other chest operations the surgeon cuts the phrenic nerve. The phrenic nerve ultimately comes from the brain and activates the diaphragm. If this happens, the patient has only about 20% of the normal amount of power to breathe.

When we breathe harder than normal, accessory muscles of breathing help with breathing in and out. Accessory muscles include the abdominal muscles and various muscle groups of the shoulders and neck. We can see athletes or asthma patients using their accessory muscles of ventilation. Just take a deep breath in and out and feel which muscles are now being used. Start by placing your hand over the upper part of your belly and breathing in and out forcefully. Next place your hand around your neck and feel the muscles contract and relax as you breathe in and out forcefully.

These two illustrations show how contraction of these muscles causes the chest to expand during inhalation. Remember, during resting breathing exhalation is just relaxing these muscles and the air "squirts" back out without effort. Labored breathing may include use of abdominal muscles to push the air out. Think about playing a trumpet or singing and using abdominal muscles to control exhalation.

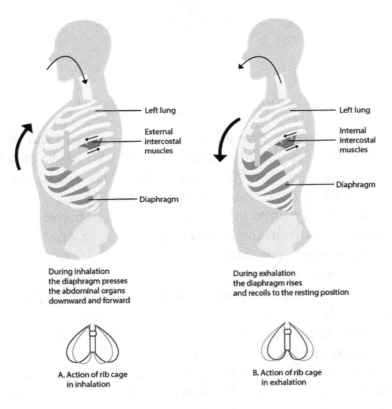

Left lung

External intercostal muscles

Diaphragm

During inhalation the diaphragm presses the abdominal organs downward and forward

Left lung

Internal intercostal muscles

Diaphragm

During exhalation the diaphragm rises and recoils to the resting position

A. Action of rib cage in inhalation

B. Action of rib cage in exhalation

Illustration of Rib Cage Action

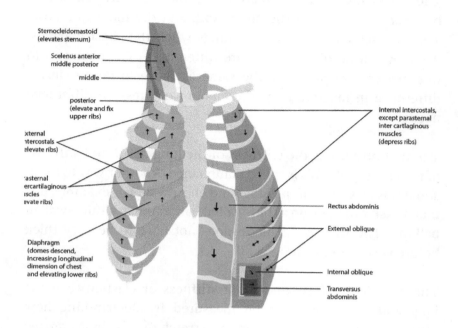

Sternocleidomastoid
(elevates sternum)

Scelenus anterior
middle posterior

middle

posterior
(elevate and fix
upper ribs)

xternal
ntercostals
elevate ribs)

·asternal
ercartilaginous
ıscles
evate ribs)

Diaphragm
(domes descend,
increasing longitudinal
dimension of chest
and elevating lower ribs)

Internal intercostals,
except parasternal
inter cartlaginous
muscles
(depress ribs)

Rectus abdominis

External oblique

Internal oblique

Transversus
abdominis

Illustration of Respiratory Muscle Actions

Work of Breathing (WOB)

WOB is primarily a matter of how much of our body's energy we spend breathing, and what obstacles we are trying to overcome. It is easy to visualize the difference in the amount of work we do in order to breathe when we are sitting watching TV versus hiking up a steep hill.

The force involved in breathing is the pressure difference between the inside of the chest wall, and the mouth or nose. This is what sucks air into the lungs when the chest expands. Air moves according to pressure differences. The obstacles to this process are normally the same as those in illness, just a difference in magnitude or the amount of pressure difference needed.

The first obstacle is the stiffness of the lung tissue and stiffness of the chest wall. This is called compliance. Another way to think about it is elasticity of the lungs and chest wall. For example, it is much easier to blow up a thin-walled balloon than a thick-walled balloon. The wall of a balloon does not have to be very thick before we can't blow it up at all.

The compliance (the amount of stiffness or elasticity) of the lung and chest wall can be measured by determining how much pressure it takes to open and stretch out the lungs during inspiration. In other words, how hard it is to get a tidal volume into the lungs. It is a very simple measurement and should be measured on all patients on ventilators. As can be easily imagined if the lungs become stiff from inflammation (swelling), injury or fibrotic changes, it is very difficult to get a breath. Likewise, if the chest wall is stiff from tight bandages around the chest, a swollen abdomen pushing up against the diaphragm, or muscle spasms from a seizure, it requires more work to breathe.

The second obstacle to breathing is resistance to airflow through the airways from the atmosphere to the functional lung tissue. This includes every air passage from the nose or mouth to the terminal bronchiole. Keep in mind that anything that makes the airway smaller makes it a lot harder to breathe. Please see the diagram below. Airway resistance increases are primarily caused by problems that decrease the diameter of the air passages. This is best described by Poiseuille (a Frenchman in the 1800s) who put forth the idea in the following mathematical equation. By the way, it looks intimidating, but it is not too bad. If you are not mathematically inclined, look at what each of the letters represent and picture it in your mind. It is just a tube with air blowing through it. The narrower the tube the harder it is to blow the air through.

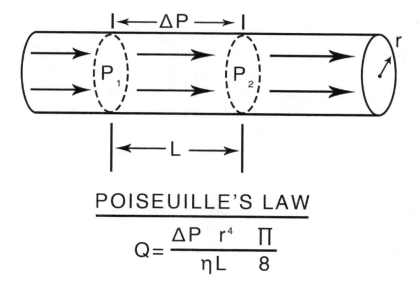

POISEUILLE'S LAW

$$Q = \frac{\Delta P \; r^4}{\eta L} \; \frac{\Pi}{8}$$

Where Q = airflow, P1 and P2 are pressures at each end of the airway, r = the radius of the airway, n = viscosity of air, L = length of the airway and 8 is a constant value as is "n".

The thing of real interest in this application of Poiseuille's Law is the inverse relationship between airway resistance and changes in the radius of the conducting tube. If we rearrange the equation

above and combine pressure/airflow which is airway resistance
"R" (cmH$_2$O/Liter/sec.), and get rid of the constants, we get

$$R = L/r4$$

Next let's get rid of "L". It is obvious to anyone that it will be
harder to blow air down a longer tube than a shorter tube. So,
resistance to airflow has mostly to do with the radius or diameter
of the tube.

We are left with the fascinating relationship between airway
resistance (R) and airway radius (r) is this: because radius is to
the 4th power, every time the radius of the airway is decreased
by half; the resistance to breathing is increased 16 times. Even
this would not be so exciting if there weren't so many factors
that can cause the airway radius in the lungs to decrease by half.
For example, bronchial muscle spasm, excessive mucus or other
secretions, inflammation or swelling, blood clots, a bronchial
tumor, or scar tissue. Sometimes, it is simply the medical
professionals providing an artificial airway of a radius too small
for reasonable breathing. The latter happens in numerous ways
more often than necessary and is never desirable.

Bottom line is anything that makes the airway smaller makes it a
lot harder to breathe.

Heart and Circulation Are Part of "Respiration"

A quick look at a normal heart anatomy will help understand much about using ventilators because the heart and lungs are so dependent on each other.

As mentioned before, the lungs are an air pump bringing air inside the body to meet up with the blood and provide oxygen and get rid of carbon dioxide from the blood. The blood is pumped by the heart around to the body and back to the lungs. The heart is actually two pumps working together. On the left side of the heart or left heart, the powerful left ventricle pumps blood to the whole body. The right heart pumps in unison with the left heart and only has to pump the blood a short distance to the lungs. It's like a figure 8 with all the blood going around two different circles each time. It is easy to see that if either side of the heart gets weak from a heart attack it is going to back up blood coming back from the other side. Both sides have to pump together and keep up with each other.

In the diagram below the heart is facing us, so the left side of the heart with red blood and more muscular walls is on the right in the diagram. The right heart getting depleted blood back from the body is blue blood and on the left in diagram. Be sure to note the directions of the arrows.

We need to keep the fact that the heart is the next step in respiration and will keep showing up in explanations of different kinds of respiratory failure.

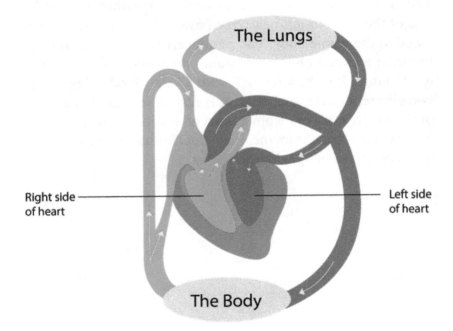

Respiratory Failure - "Not Normal Breathing"

Failure to breathe normally gets our attention. The slogan of the American Lung Association captures this concept very well, "When you can't breathe nothing else matters." Feeling a little short of breath is scary. Being unable to breathe at all is terrifying, but only for a few minutes if nothing is done. Probably that is why it is terrifying; because, those who weren't terrified were not around to reproduce.

Respiratory failure means the patient <u>cannot breathe</u> well enough. Medical professionals should never give "respiratory failure" as the only reason a patient is on a ventilator. Even small children can tell when someone <u>cannot breathe</u>. Medical professionals should explain the problem much more specifically and fully if they understand the patient's problem and care to communicate. For example, the physician comes out of the emergency room and explains to the family, "Your loved one went into respiratory failure and we had to place them on a ventilator." The family might reply, "She was breathing well when we brought her in here, please tell us something more specific, so we can understand the problem." Health care providers tend to oversimplify and minimize; especially, if they don't know what is going on.

Respiratory failure takes two very simple forms, as described before, failure for the good air to go in and failure of the bad air to get out. Although these two processes are closely related, they are quite different and require quite different interventions to reverse. We call the former "oxygenation problems" and the latter "ventilatory failure". Let's look at each more closely.

Oxygenation Failure

Everyone knows that we cannot survive without an adequate supply of oxygen. This is what suffocation is all about. It is generally accepted that after 4 – 6 minutes without oxygen irreversible brain death begins. The tissues most vulnerable to damage and malfunction due to lack of oxygen are the heart, kidneys and brain, all vital organs.

Words associated with low oxygen are hypoxia (low oxygen), hypoxemia (low oxygen in the blood) and anoxia (no oxygen). Anoxia is not often used in this context; because, we do not see a complete absence of oxygen in living human beings.

Oxygenation of the human body is quite well understood. Oxygen is breathed or ventilated into the lungs where it crosses through the alveolocapillary membrane into the blood. Oxygen in the blood is primarily carried by hemoglobin molecules in red blood cells. Oxygenated blood is pumped to all parts of the body.

To assess the adequacy of oxygenation we must look at several factors.

First, is enough oxygen getting into the blood? Partial pressure of oxygen in the arterial blood (P_aO_2), and oxygen saturation of hemoglobin in the blood (S_pO_2) measure this. We often hear of S_pO_2 because pulse oximeters are becoming more popular over-the-counter or even in smart watches.

Normal P_aO_2 = 80 -100 mmHg. We don't like it to go below 60 mmHg. Don't worry about the term "partial pressure." For our purposes it is just a unit of measurement of the amount of oxygen dissolved in the plasma of arterial blood. The glossary of this book contains a more detailed definition if you are curious.

Normal S_pO_2 = 95-99%; we don't like to see it go much lower than 89%. This is the percentage of the hemoglobin in the blood that is carrying oxygen. This is a little more important to understand as the pulse oximeter to measure S_pO_2 is available over-the-counter in drugstores and on the internet. It is also important because the hemoglobin in the red blood cells carry most of the oxygen.

The efficiency of the process of oxygenation of the blood is one of the more complicated concepts in mechanical ventilation. It is covered in depth in Chapter 6. Briefly, the efficiency of the respiratory unit, air sacs and pulmonary capillaries, can be calculated or estimated by looking at the oxygen needs of the depleted blood coming back to the respiratory unit. If we compare this need to the amount of oxygen that ends up in the refreshed blood going out to the heart and body, we can get an idea how well this is working. At the same time, we must keep in mind the amount of oxygen available, or that might have been available in the ideal alveolus. This efficiency measure is called right to left intrapulmonary shunt fraction. In other words, it tells us how much of the total amount of deoxygenated blood pumped by the right heart to the lungs is not coming in contact with well-aerated alveoli. Or vice versa, how much oxygen depleted blood is coming in and matching with well-aerated alveoli.

Here is a useful analogy. Imagine a line of buckets going at an even speed under a pipe pouring out water. If the buckets are empty, and there is plenty of water flowing from the source the buckets should all get filled up on the way through. If the buckets are empty coming in for filling and something is cutting off the water flow, the buckets will only get partially filled. Here we could look at the buckets coming out and estimate how badly the water is being dammed up. Like most analogies this is not perfect because the oxygen depleted blood coming in from the body has some varying amount of oxygen on board and is looking for a fill up. So, we have to look at all three factors to estimate efficiency of the respiratory unit.

Second, is there enough hemoglobin in the blood, (Hb)? This is a regularly measured laboratory test taken from a patient blood sample. Normal hemoglobin is 12 -15 ml/dl.

Third, is there enough blood being pumped around? This can be measured by heart rate and blood pressure, or cardiac output in liters per minute. The efficiency of circulation can be calculated.

Fourth, is the amount of oxygen available adequate to meet body needs? This can be assessed by looking at the amount of oxygen remaining in mixed venous blood returning to the heart from the body, mixed venous oxygen saturation, S_vO_2 and arterial-venous oxygen difference, avDO$_2$. That is, how much oxygen was left over after the body took what it needed. It usually leaves the blood about 75% full, $S_vO_2 = 75\%$. If it gets below $S_vO_{2=}$ 50 %, it is a serious problem. These measurements are rather difficult and are not routinely measured. However, if a ventilator patient has a "Swan-Ganz" or pulmonary artery catheter, these measurements can and should be taken. This complex topic is discussed more fully in Chap 6.

Oxygenation problems can be caused by the breakdown of this chain of events at any point. For example, the oxygen may not get breathed into the lungs, oxygen in the lungs may not get into the blood, the blood may not contain enough hemoglobin, the heart may not be pumping the blood around or the blood vessels are shut down and little blood is getting to the body tissues. Respiratory care providers must assess all of these factors in order to understand a patient's oxygenation status.

One question that often arises is: "Why do we examine arterial blood gas values to assess function of the lungs?" We measure partial pressure of arterial oxygen and carbon dioxide, P_aO_2 and P_aCO_2. The reason is that the blood leaving the lungs is full of oxygen and reduced in carbon dioxide. It goes back to the powerful left side of the heart and is pumped out to all parts of the body through arteries. Arteries are the vessels where pulse and blood pressure are measured. We want to look at this blood to assess the lungs because it has just come from the lungs. Most laboratory blood samples are taken from low pressure veins taking spent blood on its way back to the heart. Venous blood from the arm would not help us very much for lung assessment.

A mechanical ventilator can only support or treat the first few steps of oxygenation problems. By far the most common and important oxygenation problem in ventilator patients is oxygen getting from the lungs into the blood. The functional problem here is that used venous blood from the body comes back to the right side of the heart and gets pumped through the lungs without coming in contact with functional lung tissue, right to left intrapulmonary shunt.

Examples of oxygenation problems for which a mechanical ventilator might be used:

	Problem (pathology)	Cause (etiology)
ARDS (Acute Respiratory Distress Syndrome)	fluid in spaces between the air sacs and capillaries; breakdown or thickening of the alveolocapillary membrane.	Shock, infection of blood or lungs, chemical inhalation, inhalation of fresh or salt water, back pressure from left heart failure
Pneumonia	Infection filling the air sacs with puss	Virus, bacteria, fungus
Pulmonary edema	Plasma from the blood pouring into the air sacs	Near-drowning, IV fluid overload
Congestive heart failure	Plasma from the blood pouring into the air sacs	Left heart failure backing blood up in the lungs
Pulmonary emphysema	Walls of air sacs rupture and become fibrotic	Cigarette smoking, occasionally other causes
Chronic bronchitis	Airway inflammation	Cigarette smoking, vaping
RDS (Respiratory Distress Syndrome) of the neonate	fluid spaces between the air sacs and capillaries	Immature lungs; pre-mature birth
Hypoventilation	Inadequate supply of fresh air	Ventilatory failure

Ventilators can supply higher concentrations of oxygen and apply expiratory pressure to the chest to help with oxygenation.

Ventilatory Failure

Ventilatory failure is different from oxygenation problems, but there is some overlap. Our body keeps the CO_2 level just right by "washing" the CO_2 out of our lungs with fresh air each breath. We do this by matching our minute volume with our metabolism. The CO_2 is constantly accumulating because CO_2 production is the result of normal body metabolism, i.e., cellular respiration. Circulating blood brings the CO_2 from all over the body back to the lungs to diffuse out of the blood into the lungs. We usually need to inhale and exhale about 3 – 5 quarts of air each minute to wash CO_2 out to an appropriate level. Breathing 12 – 20 times a minute, we are able to do this. Thus, the level of CO_2 in our body is directly related to the air moving in and out of our lungs, or minute volume of our lungs.

$$(P_aCO_2 \sim \text{minute volume})$$

Anything that decreases minute volume without decreasing metabolism or CO_2 production will result in ventilatory failure. When $PaCO_2$ rises above 45 mmHg, it is called "hypoventilation" (low ventilation) and is to some degree ventilatory failure. A little hypoventilation is uncomfortable; we feel short of breath. With severe hypoventilation, very little breathing is terrifyingly miserable. Apnea, no breathing, becomes fatal rapidly.

Ventilatory failure has four (4) general origins. They are increased airway resistance (clogged or narrowed bronchial tubes), decreased lung thoracic compliance (stiff lungs or chest wall) and/or lack of respiratory drive (no signal from the brain to breathe), and respiratory muscle weakness.

The only other important aspect of ventilation is "wasted" ventilation. A certain amount of this occurs normally. For example, the trachea (windpipe) and bronchial tubes do not allow CO_2 and O_2 to cross their relatively thick walls to exit or enter the blood; therefore, the air we work to move through those tubes, although necessary, is considered "wasted" ventilation. The medical term for wasted ventilation is "deadspace ventilation". Normal deadspace ventilation of the airways is about 15-40% of the tidal volume. When blood vessel disease in the lungs does not allow blood flow to the functional air sacs, these areas that exchange CO_2 and O_2 become deadspace ventilation.

This sounds complicated. Simply put, the CO_2 keeps building up in the blood even though plenty of air is going in and out of the lungs. So, the patient looks like they are breathing adequately or even breathing excessively; however, the CO_2 cannot get out of the blood. In this case the CO_2 rises up out of 35 – 45 mmHg. range in spite of rapid, deep breathing. Deadspace ventilation is very difficult for medical professionals to measure but happens quite frequently. The easy way to figure this out is if the patient is breathing more than 4 – 6 liters/min. to keep CO_2 normal, or the patient has a high CO_2 in the face of normal or excessive minute volume, then there is likely increased deadspace ventilation. The diagram of a respiratory unit below shows a pulmonary capillary on the right side clotted with blood and no blood going to the alveolus. Because it is being ventilated it is deadspace ventilation or wasted ventilation. The diagram also shows anatomic deadspace ventilation that occurs in large airways that are not in contact with the blood, and also mechanical tubing that could be added onto the patient's endotracheal tube. Anatomic deadspace is normal. Alveolar deadspace is the problem. Mechanical deadspace should be minimized in the ventilator circuit.

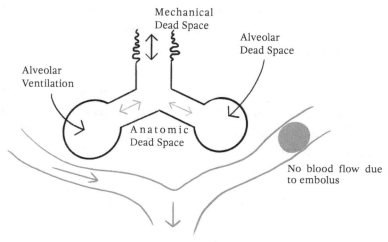

The question might come up about exhaled CO_2 build up in the air or rebreathing our exhaled air. The CO_2 concentration in the atmosphere is almost zero as far as breathing is concerned. There is more argon (0.90%) in the atmosphere than CO_2 (0.03%). Both are less than 1%. In fact, exhaled air is used in mouth-to-mouth resuscitation to save lives. Neither of these issues, although logical questions, are worth further consideration in a discussion of mechanical ventilation.

Of the four reasons people end up in ventilatory failure, perhaps the easiest to understand is lack of respiratory drive. Simply put, the brain is not sending a message to the respiratory muscles to tell them to breathe. There are numerous reasons for this to occur, for example, drug overdose, brain stroke, head trauma, too much sedation or pain killers. A too frequent example is a patient after surgery that has an IV pump for pain control. The patient is pushing the button constantly to get more pain killer, and it starts to depress the respiratory centers in the brain. The patient then stops breathing and hopefully the hospital staff notice this in time and the patient is quickly intubated, placed on a ventilator, and given medication to reverse the excessive pain medicine. It is entirely possible this patient might come off the ventilator in a couple hours and have their future doses of pain meds reduced.

Finally, the respiratory muscles can become weak and cannot respond to the call of normal ventilation. This is most commonly caused by neuromuscular diseases or perhaps malnutrition. Just because a patient is on a ventilator in an intensive care unit does not mean that they are well nourished. Inadvertent malnutrition in ICU is much less these days when nutritionists are part of the ICU team.

Examples of ventilatory failure follow:

	Problem (pathology)	Cause (etiology)
Asthma	Increased work of breathing	Swollen bronchial tubes squeezed by muscle spasms
Anesthesia	No stimulus to breathe	Sedation of the brain and/ or paralysis of muscles
Upper airway obstruction	Increased work of breathing	Tumor, swollen or flaccid soft tissues in the airway
Lower airway obstruction	Increased work of breathing	Tumor, fibrotic tissues, excessive thick mucus
Pulmonary emphysema	Increased work of breathing	Cigarette smoking, occasionally other causes
Chronic bronchitis	Increased work of breathing	Cigarette smoking, vaping
Morbid obesity	Increased work of breathing	Abdominal contents pushing against diaphragm
Chest trauma	Increased work of breathing Decreased mechanics	Surgery, automobile crash, other physical violence
Head trauma	No stimulus to breathe	Surgery, automobile crash, other physical violence

Mysathenia gravis	Weak respiratory muscles	Abnormal neurotransmitters
Foreign body in airway	Increased work of breathing	Choking on food or other objects
Broken neck	No transmission of the stimulus to breathe	Automobile crash, other physical violence
Sedative drug overdose	No stimulus to breathe	Sedation of the brain
Stroke/ Intracranial bleed	No stimulus to breathe	High blood pressure, cigarette smoking, etc.

CHAPTER 3

The Machines

They are called ventilators, "the breathing machine", or respirators. They really do little more than ventilate the lungs and provide life support for a person until underlying medical problems can be reversed. Mechanical ventilators are life support equipment. They are possibly the most dramatic or impressive piece of life support equipment in common use. If you walk up to a patient's bedside in an intensive care unit (ICU) you will notice the machine rhythmically blowing air into the patient. It is somehow fascinating. If you are not careful you may even find yourself breathing in rhythm with the machine.

The ventilators pictured below represent some of the most sophisticated machines in the world. The two machines on the pedestals are microprocessor-controlled and are fully loaded with automation and advanced features to help the clinician in every aspect of ICU ventilator care. The smaller ventilator on the table is the Airon Medical, pNeuton ventilator chosen by the U.S. government, Ford and GE Healthcare to make tens of thousands to solve the ventilator shortage caused by the COVID-19 pandemic. The pNeuton is a pneumatic ventilator and does not require electricity.

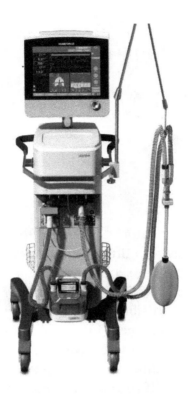

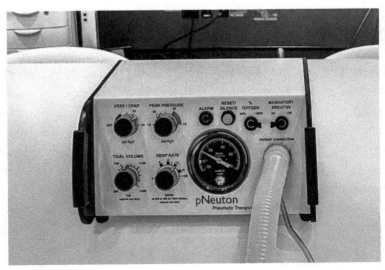

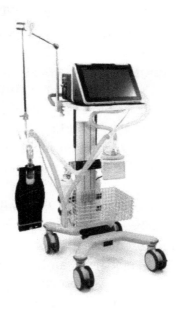

Ventilators are absolutely necessary for the patient who needs one to stay alive, except in very unusual circumstances. Mechanical ventilators have very little therapeutic capability and create conditions for many complications. They are probably best viewed as a necessary evil, and their necessity should be carefully assessed from not only a medical perspective, but also, and most importantly, from a social, ethical perspective.

The use of, and the need for, mechanical ventilation must be assessed and reassessed frequently. The respiratory therapist, intensivist and ICU nurse will be assessing the need for the ventilator routinely every few hours, and every time the patient has a major change in condition that affects the ventilator. At least once a day the patient is given a chance to see if they can breathe on their own (spontaneous breathing trial). The spontaneous breathing trial may be canceled if the patient is so critically ill and fragile that this procedure will likely cause grave danger. The words "grave danger" are being used appropriately.

Highly automated ventilators will assess the need for many aspects of the patient's need for the ventilator as often as breath-to-breath and in some cases within a single breath. These microprocessor-based machines can make their own setting changes and either add or subtract life support functions according to an embedded computer protocol.

This book is about ICU ventilators. ICU ventilators have a great number of settings to breathe the patient appropriately. ICU ventilators have many monitoring functions to provide data to the ICU practitioners. They have amazing alarm and patient safety functions that often have double or triple redundancy. Triple redundancy means if a first-line alarm fails a back-up alarm will come on, if the backup alarm fails, a third system is in place to keep the patient safe. Failure of an ICU ventilator is catastrophic, and systems are in place to support the patient should that highly unlikely event ever occur.

There are much less sophisticated ventilators for other uses. The simplest "ventilator" is like a fireplace bellows or an air mattress pump. They both pump air. As described in the earlier chapters, ventilators blow or push air into the lungs using positive pressure from outside the patient. They have an exhalation valve that closes while the machine blows air and into the lungs. The exhalation valve opens on exhalation, allowing the air to come back out of the patient passively by the recoil of the respiratory muscles and the chest wall. Ventilators do not suck.

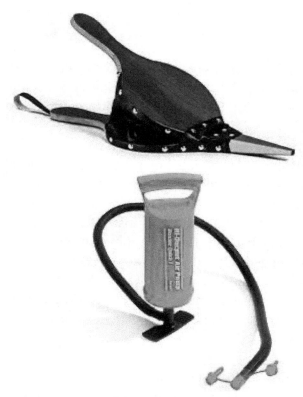

At every ventilator patient bedside is a simple, manual resuscitator for hand-powered ventilation in case of any type of power failure or in-operation malfunction of the ICU ventilator. A manual resuscitator is pictured below.

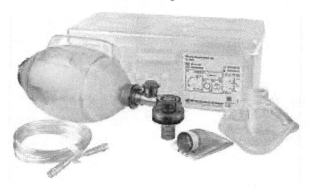

Power Supply

Ventilators are portable machines that are powered by electricity and need a continuous supply of high-pressure air and oxygen. Some ventilators are powered by pneumatics or just compressed air or oxygen.

The supply of electricity must be reliable. ICUs have generators backing up electrical supply via special color-coded red outlets. A ventilator should not be plugged into a regular electrical outlet if red outlets are available. In addition, most ICU ventilators have an internal battery back-up that will come on instantly if the ventilator is unplugged or there is a power outage. Initiation of the internal battery is accompanied by audible and visible alarms. So, everyone present knows which electrical supply source is in use. The internal batteries have a wide variation in battery life but usually last for 30 mins to 4 hours.

The supply of high-pressure oxygen is usually from huge liquid oxygen tanks placed outside the medical center. The liquid oxygen evaporates and pushes the resulting gaseous oxygen into the hospital through a special plumbing system. These liquid systems are highly reliable and do not depend on electricity. Oxygen can also be supplied from compressed oxygen cylinders when needed. These cylinders look like scuba tanks or welders' gas tanks. Depending on the size of the oxygen tank it can last from 15 to 20 mins to several hours; however, someone has to be diligent in monitoring oxygen tank pressure and having back-up oxygen available. Oxygen can also be supplied by oxygen concentrators that sieve oxygen out of the air. Use of oxygen concentrators for ventilators is unusual and does depend on electricity.

Most ventilators have a pressurized air supply either from large hospital-based air compressors, portable air compressors or high-speed turbines within the ICU ventilator itself. Of course, the air supply must be reliable like electricity and oxygen. Some newer ventilators have high-speed turbines that provide very reliable high-pressure air source.

Please note that the common usage of the words, "unplugging life support" refers to ventilators specifically. If a patient is to be removed from the ventilator for whatever reason, the ventilator is first disconnected from the patient's airway, not by pulling the electrical plug. Then, the ventilator may be turned off using the power switch. As described in the previous paragraph, if the ventilator is just unplugged most of them will just keep ventilating with the back-up battery.

Internal Ventilator Controls

Internally ventilators are integrated, mechanical, pneumatic, electronic, and microprocessor systems. These systems serve two primary functions. First, they provide and control gas to breathe the patient. Second, they monitor the patient and ventilator function.

Automated ventilators have another level of embedded control and decision-making systems. This makes ventilator engineering and maintenance complicated. Added to this is the criticality of their function. This is not a machine you want breaking down and needing repair frequently. They must be extremely reliable and need infrequent maintenance. Ventilators go through a rigorous approval process by the FDA before going to market.

Between different patients, the ventilator is disinfected, and all single-patient use parts including the entire breathing circuit are replaced. After reassembly and prior to the use on another patient the ventilator is connected to an artificial lung and an operational verification procedure (OVP) is conducted checking all important ventilator functions and alarm functions. The OVP is documented and signed for future reference.

Trip through the ventilator

Let us follow gaseous flow through a typical ventilator/patient system. Compressed oxygen and compressed air from wall outlets come into the ventilator through a water trap and filter. These supply gases should be completely dry (close to 0% humidity) and clean. The pressure is 50 pounds per square inch above atmospheric pressure.

The ventilator reduces this pressure with an internal regulator to some working pressure. The two gases go to a gas mixer. This allows the respiratory therapist to choose any oxygen concentration between pure air at 21% oxygen (79% nitrogen) and pure 100% oxygen. The mixed gas is then precisely metered out to the patient through microprocessor-controlled valves. Some of these valves are pristinely controllable by the microprocessor making very fine adjustments to the gas flow to the patient in a matter of milliseconds. Other machines have less sophisticated solenoid valves that simply snap open or closed on electronic signals. The gas going to the patient exits the cabinet of the machine through a bacteria/viral filter, and a humidifier and enters a disposable plastic tubing called a patient breathing circuit.

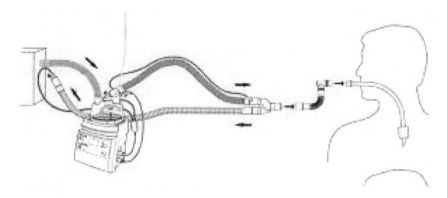

Illustration of the patient breathing circuit with a heated humidifier

The breathing circuit has an inspiratory limb (hose) taking gas to the patient and an expiratory limb (hose) returning exhaled gas to the exhalation or exhaust valve. The gas exhausted back into the room passes through one final bacteria/virus filter.

Let's go back and look more closely at certain parts of this trip through the ventilator.

The source gas is very clean. The oxygen is boiled off a bulk, liquid oxygen storage system and piped through copper pipes throughout the medical center. Air is compressed by a medical-grade air compressor at the medical center and has its own system of pipes in the hospital ceilings and walls. Both gases are filtered for bacteria and virus before entering the ventilator patient circuit. This clean gas and the correct mixture of oxygen then goes to the inspiratory valve.

The inspiratory valve that produces the patient's breath is controlled by the microprocessor. The microprocessor signals the inspiratory valve to generate a certain size breath, how often the patient gets a breath (respiratory rate), and the characteristic of the gas flow during the breath. Mechanical and software engineers program the microprocessor to offer a number of options for the user to select from the control knobs or video screen on the front of the ventilator. The valves will then deliver a set volume of gas each breath or to provide a set amount of pressure to drive the breath into the patient. The characteristic of the breath can be changed breath-to-breath or within a breath. The response time of the inspiratory valves to the microprocessor is milliseconds.

The inspiratory valve is sensitive. Sensitivity is a concept associated with the relationship between the microprocessor, the inspiratory valve and the patient. Sensitivity is the relative ease with which the patient can signal the ventilator to get a breath on demand. The sensitivity control is also called the "trigger". A more sensitive ventilator will trigger more easily when a patient initiates their own breath (spontaneous breath). Ventilators have some variation in their ability to sense the patient's breath initiation. Then it is a matter of how fast the microprocessor and inspiratory valves can respond to deliver air to the patient. This response time and how much flow or pressure is necessary to trigger a breath are measures of sensitivity. Ventilators sense either a pressure drop (pressure trigger) in the breathing circuit or the initiation of air flow (flow trigger) when the patient starts to take a spontaneous breath. The respiratory therapist can select either pressure trigger or flow trigger and the degree of work the patient is required to get a breath. Generally, the more sensitive the ventilator is to the patient the better. However, too much sensitivity can cause the ventilator to automatically provide gas flow at rapid intervals out of synchrony with patient breathing. This autocycling or "chatter" is very disturbing to the patient. Likewise, a ventilator that is not sensitive enough causes increased work of breathing for the patient, and is perceived as discomfort or struggling to get a breath, or they can't get a breath at all.

The gases traveling through the ventilator have no humidity. They have to be passed through a humidifier before reaching the patient's respiratory tract. Normally our nose and upper airways warm and humidify inspired air to 100% relative humidity at body temperature before the air gets to the functional portion of our lungs.

The humidifiers come in two quite dissimilar varieties.

First, the heated humidifier, is a container that allows warm water vapor to enter the inspiratory gas to the ventilator patient. These humidifiers must be carefully adjusted in order to provide the right amount of humidity. If the inspired gas is too dry it will dry out the secretions in the patient's airways and form hard mucus plugs. If the inspired gas is too wet, it will rain out and form puddles in the patient's circuit inspiratory limb. This can cause bubbling and vibrating and provide a medium (environment/food) for growth of infection. It is also possible that the patient can get this puddled water poured down their unprotected airway when someone drains the water out of the patient circuit the wrong direction either intentionally or while turning the patient. Water bubbling in the inspiratory limb should be minimized or eliminated. These heaters can also get too hot or too cold. Clearly, inspired gas that is too hot or too cold is not good for the patient. Many ventilator circuits have heated wires inside the hoses that maintain the gas temperature to minimize the condensation of rainout in the circuit. According to the 2012 American Association for Respiratory Care, Clinical Practice Guidelines, a maximum delivered gas temperature of 37°C (98.6° F) and 100% RH (44 mg H2O/L.) at the circuit

Y-piece is recommended. Ventilator heated humidifiers contain alarms for safe function as well as a low water supply alarm.

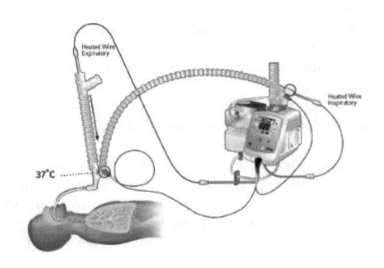

Second, there is a heat moisture exchanger (HME) which involves a physical process. It is a filter that removes heat and moisture from the patient's exhaled air and places it back into the air of the next breath going in. The HME is sometimes called an "artificial nose." HME has been compared to the nose of a camel. Apparently, camel's noses retain water from the exhaled air and put it back in the next breath.

Either type of humidifier is adequate for most patients. The advantage of the HME is cost and safety. The HME will not overheat, will not produce rain out or will not drive the staff crazy with alarms. However, the HME does not work as well for patients with very thick, sticky airway secretions, (mucus). Also, the HME can become a problem for patients with large amounts of mucus or blood coughing out of the patient circuit that clogs up the HME filter.

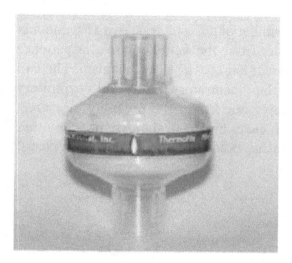

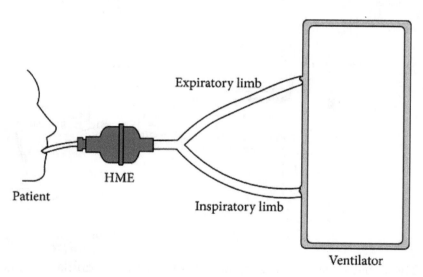

Illustration of an HME and a diagram of its place in the patient breathing circuit

Humidifiers provide warm moist gases to the lungs. Humidifiers must be monitored for proper function at frequent intervals.

The patient circuit is a number of hoses, at least two, that conduct the breath, tidal volume, from the ventilator to the patient's airway and back to the ventilator exhaust mechanism. The two main tubes are called the "inspiratory limb" and "expiratory limb". As the names imply one brings the precisely measured, pressurized, humidified, clean breath to the patient. The other dumps the patient's passive exhalation out through an exhaust valve and expiratory filter.

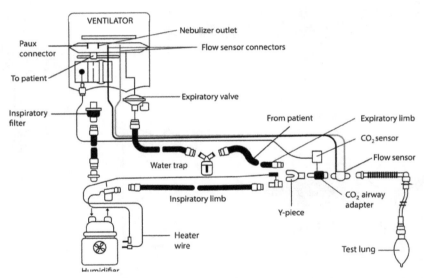

Illustration of detailed patient breathing circuit.

The exhaust valve is a very important part of a ventilator. It is a one-way valve that stays shut during the inspiratory phase of ventilation. This closes the tubing system between the patient and the atmosphere, so that the ventilator can build up pressure and push the tidal volume into the patient's lungs. After a certain amount of time or some other signal the inspiratory gas shuts off ending inspiration and the exhaust valve opens at the same time. With the open exhaust valve, the tidal volume and pressure in the patient's lungs escape out through the expiratory filter into the room. The important characteristic of the exhaust valve is that it can open quickly and widely in order to allow the patient to exhale passively and easily. A surprising additional function of the exhaust valve is that it is often held partially closed in order to trap a certain amount of pressure to hold the patient's lungs and airways open. This is called Positive End-Expiratory Pressure (PEEP) and is discussed thoroughly in Chapter 4.

The expiratory filter is a relatively simple device that filters the exhaled air before dumping it back into the atmosphere. The exhaled air out of the filter goes into the patient's room where visitors and health care workers are present and breathing. These filters are usually at least 99.99% effective. The object is to prevent the spread of infection.

The other hoses and wires in the patient circuit might include an airway pressure monitoring line, an airway temperature monitoring probe, double lines to an inspiratory and expiratory flow measuring sensor, a wire to a carbon dioxide detector, and or the pneumatic power supply to an in-line, small volume, medication nebulizer. One item that is often present is an in-line suction apparatus. This device is a long, flexible catheter that is encased in a slender plastic bag. It is connected to the hospital wall vacuum system and allows the patient caregivers to introduce the enclosed catheter into the patient's lungs and suction or aspirate secretions out of the patient's artificial and natural airways without opening the tubing system to infection. This procedure is described in Chapter 7.

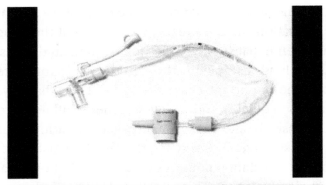

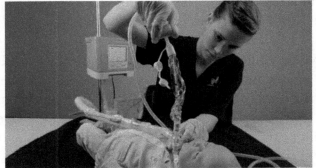

Illustrations of an in-line suction catheter and its use

The Ventilator Display Screen

The display screen is the most prominent visual feature on the front of a ventilator. On lower-end ventilators the screen may be a digital display of a few most important patient monitoring data and/or the ventilator and alarm settings. On the simplest ventilators it is just an analog pressure gauge like the one on a bicycle tire pump. On the highly sophisticated ventilators the display screen can be configured by the respiratory therapists to display whatever information is most important to the ICU ventilator patient care team. These high-end ventilators collect and show entirely too much information to be seen on one screen. So, the screens can be scrolled through to see whatever data or graphs are of the most interest. The specific data or graph images can be placed anywhere on the front screen of the ventilator for ease of use or brought into view by clicking tabs or icons. Many of the display screens are touch screens. Many of the displays can provide screenshots for documentation and /or be "frozen" to capture specific data or to take

measurements off of graphs.

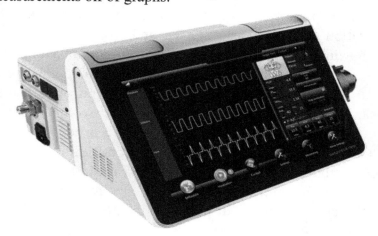

Illustration of a most sophisticated Vyaire, Bella Vista ventilator touch screen display

The screen on the Bella Vista 1000, Vyaire, above, operates very much like a smart phone providing access to ventilator settings, prediction of future change in the patient-ventilator relationship, tutorials on specialized setups, and customization of the ventilator to the specific patient and disease entity.

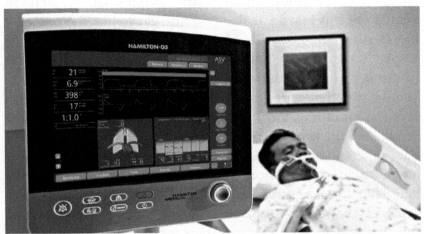

Illustration of the Hamilton Medical ventilator screen, cockpit view

The Hamilton Medical ventilators provide a main screen that is much like the cockpit of an airplane placing the most vital information where it's easiest to see, and projecting a dynamic lung showing the practitioner several most important parameters in a single glance. The Dynamic Lung is similar in concept to the Attitude Indicator in every airplane cockpit. An Attitude Indicator is a little airplane graphic in space, so the pilot can see in a glance if the plane is going up, down or to either side. In an instant the operator can get the most critical information regarding the current situation as the Dynamic Lung has the most important information regarding airway resistance and lung/thoracic compliance display prominently and clearly.

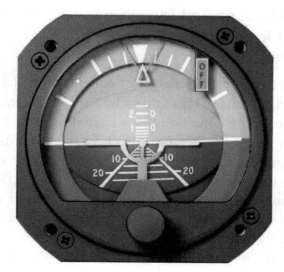

Airplane Attitude Indicator

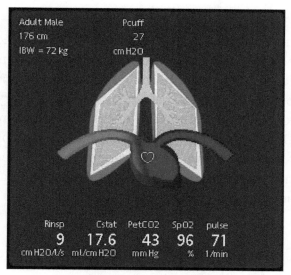

Hamilton Dynamic Lung Indicator

Data Collection and Interface to the Electronic Medical Record

The better ICU ventilators collect patient safety data and other user specified data in logs or trends. The user can quickly query what times alarm conditions have alerted the staff in the last 24 hrs. The respiratory therapist can check what ventilator settings were changed and at what time. The ventilator can also trend several monitoring functions like peak pressure, tidal volume, minute volume, expiratory resistance, compliance at the same time and choose which ones to display out of a "library" of monitored values. These can be examined over time to better understand associations between various parameters, or to see what happened prior to or during some event that happened to the patient.

Many newer ventilators can be electronically interfaced to the patient's electronic medical record. This is a great patient safety feature which among other advantages prevents human error in transcribing hundreds of data points charted everyday by the respiratory therapist. This feature can allow the Director of the ICU or Respiratory Care Department leader to look at the ventilator remotely or project the patient's display screen on the wall of a conference room for case presentation or a remote training room for educational purposes.

Devices Connecting the Ventilator to the Patient

The physical connection of the ventilator to the patient is critical.

Endotracheal tube: The most common connection of the ventilator to the patient is via an endotracheal tube through the patient's nose or mouth. The oral or nasal endotracheal tube is placed through the mouth using laryngoscope, a scope to visualize the vocal cords in the larynx (voice box). In the illustrations below you can see this tube goes through the mouth or nose, down through the larynx (voice box) to get to the trachea where the balloon (cuff) is inflated which seals against the walls of the trachea. This creates a tight seal so the high-pressure gas pumped by the ventilator will go through the endotracheal tube into the lungs rather than leak out. When an endotracheal tube is in place the patient cannot speak, eat or drink. The larger the diameter of the endotracheal tube the better the patient can breathe. (Remember Poiseuille's equation, the radius of the tube to the 4th power). Endotracheal tubes for adults range from 7.5, 8.0, 8.5, 9.0, 9.5 mm internal diameter. An endotracheal that is too small in diameter can preclude an adult to breathe on their own successfully. For example, some references state that the 7.0 mm endotracheal tube is the average size for adult women. A 7.0 mm endotracheal tube has a smaller internal diameter than a McDonald's Restaurant soda straw. It is a good ventilator patient empathy experiment to get a McDonald's straw and breath through it for a few minutes. See how you like it? If that is fun, try a regular sized drinking straw.

Correct placement of the oro/nasal endotracheal tube is very important. It is easy to insert it into the esophagus (food tube to the stomach); that is clearly going to be a disaster. It is easy to push it down too far into the right mainstem bronchus and ventilate the right lung only; that is not a good idea. When the tube is in place, multiple methods are used to determine correct placement, and they are all documented. Then it is the job of the respiratory therapist and ICU to secure the tube and document its exact placement in centimeters from the tip of the tube. This distance is usually referenced to the patient's teeth or lip. Once this is known it must be checked frequently to be sure that it is not going down deeper or coming out inadvertently. The endotracheal tube can be displaced if the patient is very active, while bathing the patient, or by the patient pulling it out with their hand when they are confused or combative.

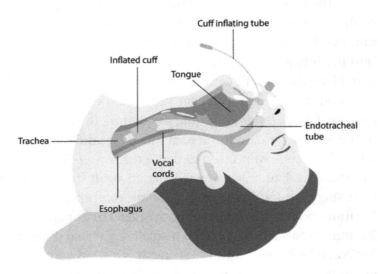

Illustration of an oral or nasal endotracheal tube and its correct placement

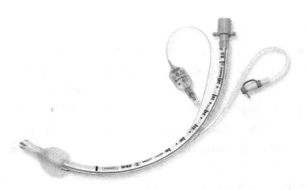

Tracheostomy tube: If the patient will be on the ventilator longer than three (3) days a tracheostomy tube connection will be considered. This is a shorter length tube introduced directly into the trachea through a surgical incision below the larynx (voice box or Adam's Apple). It has a balloon seal like the oro/nasal endotracheal tube but is more comfortable as there is no long tube going through the mouth, nose or larynx. In some cases the patient can speak, eat and drink with the tracheostomy tube in place, albeit with great difficulty.

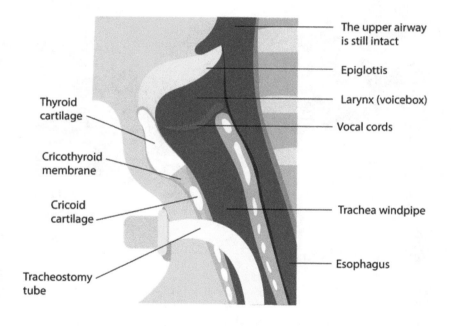

Illustration of a tracheostomy tube in place

Face Mask: The third patient ventilator connection can be a face mask. A non-invasive face mask has to have a very good seal and a special function on the ventilator that allows for leaks. The mask is strapped on the patient's face to ensure a good seal and so that it won't come off. Face mask use is called non-invasive ventilation (NIV). NIV is particularly common in the case of patients who are expected to be ventilated for only a short time or at low levels of pressure for longer times. The face mask looks uncomfortable, but does not damage the delicate tissues in the windpipe to make the airtight seal between the ventilator and patient.

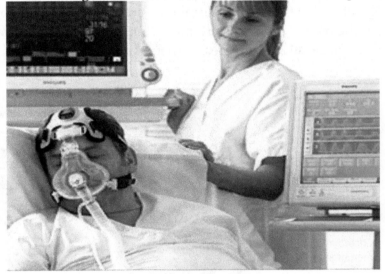

Illustration of an ICU ventilator patient with face mask connection to the ventilator

Ventilator Alarms:

The ventilator has numerous alarms. Possibly 20 or 30 conditions will activate an alarm. Some alarms are just notification of some minor discrepancy to the operator. Other alarms are signals of life-threatening emergencies. Newer model ventilators have three different alarm sounds mandated by national and international regulatory agencies. The character of each alarm, frequency, loudness and rhythm, is associated with the degree of urgency of the alarm condition. Some alarm parameters are adjustable by the respiratory therapist, others are default settings by the manufacturer.

Some general statements about alarms are necessary.

First, with this many visual (lights) and audible (sirens, beeps, bells, buzzers) alarms on the ventilator and even more alarms on ICU monitors and other ICU apparatus, there is a cacophony of alarms in the patient's room. A few are critical and life threatening, but the majority are not. These alarms are being monitored by computers as well as by the staff. The staff can often tell which alarm is sounding from a distance and may not come running every time an alarm sounds. This may be appropriate; however, in general, someone should be responding to alarms.

Second, there are at least two ways for staff to appropriately respond to an alarm. One is to correct the underlying problem or, two, the staff can silence the alarm temporarily, turn it off or readjust its limits. Most often the former is most appropriate; however, occasionally the latter is an acceptable response. Silencing or turning off the alarm can be inappropriate if not negligent if it puts the patient's well-being in jeopardy. Of course, the alarms can be ignored which is not acceptable.

There is an ICU phenomenon called "alarm fatigue" which all ICU staff must fight against. More fully automated ventilators alarm less than standard ventilators as they take care of the problem or prevent it by monitoring and adjusting to the changing patient condition. Automation can help with alarm fatigue by reducing unnecessary alarms, so ICU staff is more likely to respond promptly to remaining more appropriate alarms.

Third, if possible, it should be communicated to the patient that alarms are a normal part of the ICU environment, and that they are for the patient's benefit. The patient's visitors should also be warned not to freak out when alarms are going off. It is appropriate to ask the staff questions about alarms.

Let's look briefly at the different types of alarms starting with more critical alarms standard to all ventilators and moving onto less critical or less common alarms.

1. **High pressure alarm** - Probably the worst-case scenario for a ventilator patient would be for the exhaust valve to fail to open and/or the ventilator to fail to stop blowing air into the patient. In this situation the air would keep going into the patient at higher and higher pressures until something bursts. Clearly this situation is absolutely unacceptable. Most ventilators have double or triple redundancy in mechanisms to prevent this occurrence. These alarms are audible, visual and have actual pressure relief mechanisms. The high-pressure alarm is usually set about 10 cmH_2O pressure higher than the patient's normal peak inspiratory pressure. Peak inspiratory pressure is measured when the full tidal volume is in the patient's lungs. This alarm is at a very safe level, maximally about 50 – 60 cmH_2O. The primary pressure relief mechanism is usually a microprocessor-controlled valve that dumps excess pressure and air in order that the peak pressure does not exceed the alarm setting. Typically, there is a redundant microprocessor-controlled system on a different circuit board if the primary pressure relief fails. Additionally, there is an internal mechanical valve in the patient circuit set at a standard pressure that will dump should the electronic mechanisms fail.

Surprisingly the high-pressure alarm sounds often, and the primary pressure relief mechanism dumps gas volume and pressure often. The most common reason for this is that the patient coughs during the inspiratory cycle, and the airway pressure spikes up in an instant. Then a pressure relief valve opens and the high-pressure alarm sounds. Also, quite often the pressure alarm sounds when the patient establishes a breathing pattern that is out of phase with the ventilator creating a temporary high-pressure spike. Another common reason the pressure alarm sounds is that the patient bites down on the oral endotracheal and the ventilator delivers the breath against the obstruction. Another very common reason is that the patient's pulmonary secretions fill the airway, and the ventilator tries to deliver a breath against this obstruction. Basically, anything that obstructs the airway will generally cause a high-pressure alarm and gas volume dump. When this happens one of the ICU staff will suction out the endotracheal tube or do whatever else is needed to relieve the patient's cough or lack of synchrony with the ventilator.

If pressure alarms happen too often, it is not good because the patient does not get part of or perhaps any of the intended breath; so the reason for the alarm needs to be determined and corrected.

2. **Low frequency or apnea alarm** – This alarm is watching for another worst-case scenario, the patient and/or the ventilator has quit breathing. Most ventilators have apnea (no breathing) back-up systems. Should the patient not breathe in a spontaneous or assist mode or the ventilator not sense adequate breathing activity for 20 or 30 secs. apnea back-up mode will automatically start breathing at some pre-set respiratory rate and tidal volume.

3. **Low Pressure or Disconnection** – this alarm is quite frequent and of considerable importance. It usually indicates that the patient has become disconnected from

the ventilator. The most likely disconnection is where the patient breathing circuit connects to the endotracheal or tracheostomy tube. This point is often disconnected by patient care providers for various reasons or may be the point of least resistance for a patient who becomes disoriented and tries to pull the tubes out of their body. Sometimes the patient becomes disconnected when turning the patient during medical procedures or bathing. Needless to say that clinicians are very careful to avoid disconnections.

4. **High/Low tidal volume alarm** – high tidal volume alarm is almost unnecessary because this is seldom a problem and would likely generate a high-pressure alarm described above. Low tidal volume is a very serious and common alarm condition.

The first problem here is if the patient is breathing spontaneously with the ventilator, and the patient's tidal volumes are getting smaller-to-inadequate. This is not good because they can get atelectasis (lung collapse), ·and/or not breathe enough to eliminate carbon dioxide.

The second common low tidal volume problem is that the patient/ventilator system has developed a leak. Leaks commonly occur around the endotracheal tube cuff. Leaks can occur anywhere else in the ventilator circuit including connections between any tubes and adapters, in the humidifier, or rarely, inside the ventilator.

Another most unhappy source of leaks is inside the patient's lungs. If the patient develops a tear in the airway or lung parenchyma (functional part of the lung), the positive pressure generated by the ventilator will push air out through the tear or hole. This will cause an air pocket to develop in the patient's chest. This is generally a situation of concern or great concern. Surgical placement of a chest tube will be required immediately or very quickly. This condition is called a pneumothorax. This condition is not uncommon and often the leak heals, and the chest tube is removed without incidence.

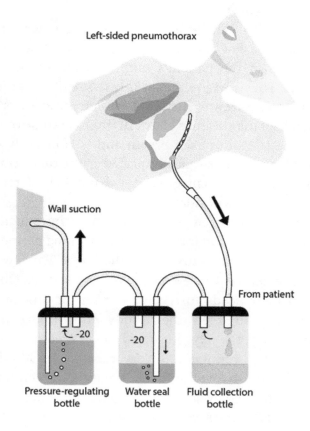

Left-sided pneumothorax

Wall suction

From patient

-20

-20

Pressure-regulating bottle

Water seal bottle

Fluid collection bottle

Illustration of a pneumothorax being drained of air and fluid with a chest tube connected to vacuum

At other times pneumothorax produces immediate, disastrous results. The immediate disaster is that a large amount of the tidal volume leaks out of the lung into the chest and collapses the leaking lung. Since the tidal volume is pressurized this can pressurize the leaking side of the chest and push on the heart and the other lung causing tension pneumothorax and cardiopulmonary failure. This can be a life-threatening emergency in a matter of a few minutes. A longer-term disaster caused by leaks in the patient's lung is called bronchopleural fistula. This is where the leaking tissue does not heal and forms a passageway (fistula) between the airways and the outside of the patient's chest. In this case some of the tidal volume leaks out each breath and is constantly drained out through the surgically placed chest tube. Obviously, this situation is dangerous for a number of reasons in addition to loss of tidal volume.

5. **High/Low Oxygen** – This alarm is infrequent. High oxygen is not good for a person over a long period of time and causes oxygen toxicity of the lungs. The low oxygen alarm is set 5 – 10% below the oxygen setting. Obviously, the patient needs to receive the set amount of oxygen necessary to keep their body functioning properly. Fortunately, the oxygen supply to the medical center and thus to the ventilator is very reliable. In addition, the ventilators have very reliable accurate oxygen mixers (+ 2%) monitored by accurate oxygen analyzers (+/- 2 - 3%).

6. **Low PEEP** – Positive End Expiratory Pressure (PEEP) is one of the few aspects of mechanical ventilation that is therapeutic; therefore, we want to know constantly that it is not below the level prescribed and set.

7. **High/Low minute volume** – this alarm is not of immediate importance; however, over time minute volume over or

under that determined to be appropriate to the patient's CO_2 production and elimination needs to be addressed.

8. **High/Low Temperature** – This ventilator humidifier alarm is set very closely to ideal body temperature of 37 degrees Centigrade or 98.6 degrees Fahrenheit. If the inspired air temperature becomes too hot it can carry too much humidity or conceivably burn the patient internally. If the air becomes too cold, it will not transport an adequate amount of humidity and the patient's airway and secretions will dry out. This latter situation is also important as dried secretions can obstruct and even plug up the airways and give the patient a serious set- back.

9. **Low water** – If the humidifier runs out of water the airway secretions will become dry very rapidly and possibly the temperature will become hot.

10. **I:E ratio** - for each breath we usually want the inspiratory time to expiratory time ratio to be less than 1:1, ideally 1:2 or 1:3. This means that the passive exhalation by the patient will have enough time to empty the previous breath before the machine or patient initiates the next breath.

When the patient does not have time to exhale, air gets trapped in their lungs' breath to breath. This trapped air is difficult to quantify and is generally considered harmful. The pressure generated by the trapped air is called auto-PEEP or inadvertent PEEP and is undesirable, difficult to measure, and sometimes difficult to avoid. We do not have an auto-PEEP alarm, so it is only by excellent assessment by the respiratory care providers that this quantity is measured, and steps are taken to reduce or remove it. Further discussion of auto-PEEP is in Chapter 6.

Finally, sometimes it is a good strategy to inverse the I:E ratio. This is where the ventilator holds inspiration longer than exhalation. In this case the physician will specifically order an I:E ratio > 1:1, perhaps 2:1 or 3:1. This is not frequently done; however, it may be a technique that is underutilized. Further discussion of inverse I:E ratio is in Chapter 6.

11. **High frequency** – An excessively high rate of breathing is a human response to exercise or difficulty breathing. A respiratory rate over 30 – 40/ min. is usually not sustainable. Sometimes nothing can be reasonably done to reduce a patient's high spontaneous respiratory rate. Other times adjusting the ventilator or medical interventions may be in order.

12. **Power disconnection** – the alarms signals that the ventilator has become unplugged from electricity, oxygen or medical compressed air, or that one of these power sources has failed. It is quite uncommon that this alarm sounds. Many ventilators have built-in battery back-up for electricity, and some have attached air compressors or built-in turbines to provide gas pressure.

13. **Ventilator inoperative** – This is definitely a bad thing! The microprocessor on the ventilator has failed, and the ventilator is probably non-functional. At this point the patient will need to be disconnected immediately and supported by hand ventilation with a manual bag/valve resuscitator. For what it is worth the bag/valve resuscitator is an adequate tool for mechanical ventilation. It is just too labor intensive and too subject to human variation for long term use.

14. **Mechanical spontaneous breathing valve** – In case of complete ventilator failure, ventilators have a mechanism that is accessible for the patient to breathe and not suffocate. This is for emergency use only and is more difficult than normal breathing which we have already determined the patient is not capable of doing. As a result, the patient

who cannot breathe well enough to start with is not very likely to do well breathing through this emergency port for more than a few seconds or minutes; however, it is "better than nothing". At least the patient would have a chance to survive. The staff will know immediately and disconnect the failed ventilator and hand ventilate with the bedside resuscitation bag. This almost never happens and would get an immediate response.

15. **Special/specific alarms** – some ventilators have unique functions that are monitored and revealed by alarm when outside certain parameters.

Price of a ventilator

The ventilator is an expensive medical device costing between $6,000 and $60,000 depending on the degree of sophistication, features, and manufacturer. Most hospitals purchase expensive "high-end" ventilators as their standard machine. They may purchase less expensive ventilators for in-house patient transport or for use in special environments like inside the Magnetic Resonance Imaging area where nothing that contains iron metal can be present.

Peripheral Equipment Related to the Ventilated Patient

Pulse Oximeter

Pulse oximeters have become common knowledge to lay people as they are often used when visiting a primary care physician or urgent care facility. They are also available in drug stores and online for purchase. A few things need to be said about the pulse oximeter. They are non-invasive and have a great technology to assess oxygenation of arterial blood without taking a blood sample. However, they work best in less critical situations and can be misleading or non-functional in full-on emergencies.

How does it work? Red light at 660nm and 940 nm is emitted from a light source on one side of the finger clip and passes through the finger to a spectrophotometer (light measuring device) on the other side of the finger clip. Oxygenated hemoglobin (HbO_2) and unoxygenated or acid hemoglobin (HHb) absorb different amounts of light at these wavelengths. The pulse oximeter is able to look only at red light being absorbed by pulsing blood. Pulsing blood is arterial blood that has most recently been oxygenated in the lungs.

The standard pulse oximeter reports both heart rate and S_pO_2 S_pO_2 = the percent of hemoglobin saturated by oxygen as measured by pulse oximeter. The percentage of the hemoglobin carrying oxygen. In healthy human beings breathing room air the arterial hemoglobin is mostly combined with oxygen.

S_pO_2 = normal value is 95 - 99%.

S_pO_2 where, S is percent saturation, p is "measured by pulse oximeter", and O_2 is oxygen.

Most pulse oximeters do not measure total hemoglobin. So, if there is very little hemoglobin as in anemia the pulse oximeter will report what percentage is oxygenated, not if there is enough hemoglobin or not.

In the case of anemia or low hemoglobin, for example if the S_pO_2 = 97% and the actual hemoglobin in the blood is 5 gm instead of 15 gm. or 1/3 of the normal amount, the patient's heart and brain could be very short of oxygen with the pulse oximeter looking perfectly normal. That is because 97% of 5 gm. of hemoglobin has oxygen, while the patient's body is starving for oxygen due to lack of enough hemoglobin carrying oxygen.

Regular pulse oximeters cannot measure abnormal hemoglobins that may be present in the blood. For example, if a person has breathed in carbon monoxide from vehicle exhaust or a slow burning fire, they may be dying of lack of oxygen due to so much abnormal carboxyhemoglobin caused by the fumes. Carboxyhemoglobin does not carry oxygen. In this case the pulse oximeter might read perfectly normal because it does not recognize the abnormal carboxyhemoglobin.

S_pO_2 does not measure oxygen delivery to the tissues. For instance, S_pO_2 = 97% and the hemoglobin in the blood is normal at 15 gm. This does not assure that the heart is pumping the blood to the body efficiently. Thus, we need to know blood pressure, pulse and, even better, cardiac output to be certain that SpO_2 = 97% is just fine.

S_pO_2 does not measure P_aCO_2 which is the measure of adequate ventilation. The patient may appear short of breath because of high carbon dioxide. The pulse oximeter may report SpO_2 = 97% when the patient is complaining of trouble breathing.

Pulse oximeters can cause people to be falsely assured of adequate oxygenation or breathing when it is actually very bad. This is unusual at home or in the family doctor's office but is much more likely in the emergency room or ICU.

We always need to look at the patient and be sure our assumptions are correct before we use the data from a pulse oximeter.

Problems with pulse oximeters are several. They don't work on cold fingers due to poor circulation because they cannot detect pulsing blood in the finger. Similarly, if the patient's blood pressure is low the pulse oximeter may not be able to detect a pulse. In the ICU, if staff is not very careful when the patient's blood pressure and cardiac output drop and the pulse oximeter isn't correct, they may increase the patient's oxygen when it was really the blood flow that was changing. Likewise, if someone is taking a blood pressure with a cuff on the same arm as the pulse oximeter, it will cut off pulsing blood flow to the finger pulse oximeter and it will temporarily fail.

Another rare occurrence is during a CPR effort. The whole resuscitation team may be looking at the monitor $S_pO_2 = 97\%$ while the heart is pumping with a good hemoglobin and assume the patient is breathing well. Then someone looking at the patient not the monitor reports the patient has stopped breathing. Again, we always need to look at the patient before making assumptions based on pulse oximetry.

Some unusual types of fingernail polish will confuse a pulse oximeter.

Pulse oximeters must be used as designed. The finger probe of the oximeter must be placed on the finger right side up. A finger probe should not be used on the patient's ear or any other part of the body that is sticking out. There are pulse oximeter sensors made for connecting to the ears and also for attaching to the patient's forehead. They need to be used as designed. Occasionally I have heard practitioners say, "Oh the finger sensor works fine on the ear. I am getting a good reading." Although they are happy with the number being reported, it may be erroneous. We don't have room for errors in medicine.

Finally, pulse oximeters are wonderful non-invasive devices to monitor patients' oxygen. In home and office use they are almost always correct. In the ICU the pulse oximeter reading has to be thoughtfully used in the context of the whole, complex patient.

Capnography - End Tidal CO_2 ($ETCO_2$)

Both end-tidal and volumetric CO_2 monitors are available as part of the ventilator, as part of the ICU nurse monitor or as stand-alone devices. End-tidal capnographs simply measure the pressure of CO_2 in the exhaled air.

End-tidal partial pressure (P_ECO_2) is a measure of carbon dioxide produced by the body. Because the sample is obtained from the exhaled air at the end of a breath, it is assumed to have come from the alveolar area of the lung where it was equilibrating with arterial carbon dioxide (P_aCO_2), or almost equal to the arterial carbon dioxide; therefore, we should be able to use it much like a blood gas result. The problem is the assumption. So even more than the pulse oximeter, we have to think critically about what we are seeing on the graph and digital readout of the capnograph.

The body processes that change P_ECO_2 are similar to those that change P_aCO_2, these are minute volume and metabolism. So, capnography with P_ECO_2 can be used to noninvasively monitor effectiveness of ventilation, and changes in metabolism without drawing an arterial blood sample.

Normal values:

$P_ECO_2 = 30 - 40$ mmHg.

Where P is partial pressure, E is end-tidal, and CO_2 is carbon dioxide.

P_ECO_2 is normally $3 - 5$ mmHg. less than P_aCO_2.

When P_ECO_2 is accurate and much lower than P_aCO_2 these numbers can be used to estimate the amount of ventilation that is going to air sacs that do not have adequate blood supply. This is called wasted ventilation or deadspace ventilation. When this happens, it can be represented by deadspace volume to tidal volume ratio (V_D/V_T). Any type of pulmonary embolism (blood clot, air bubble or fat globule) could cut off blood supply to ventilated air sacs. This is not uncommon among ventilator patients.

When using the capnograph several considerations must be made before accepting the reported result. The capnograph will report a single number to the device screen, as well as a graph of CO_2 against time. Both must be analyzed before acceptance of the single digital value reported on the screen. It only takes a moment.

Steps to success with $ETCO_2$ understanding and interpretation include checking for plateau, Phase III, on the waveform, and whenever possible correlate with the P_aCO_2 from an arterial blood sample. See the typical $ETCO_2$ tracing below.

The waveform has a plateau and is probably accurate. Look at the illustration right and see Phase III. That is the plateau.

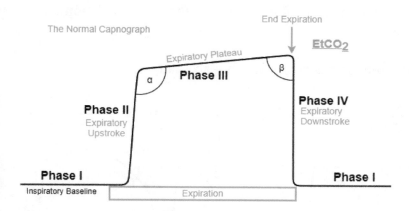

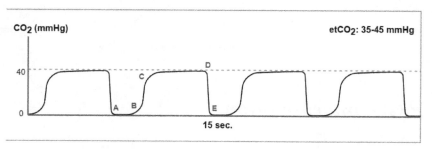

Illustration of a normal capnograph waveform

Below is an ETCO$_2$ tracing without plateau. It is missing a Phase III. It moves from early exhalation, Phase II, directly to Phase IV and the next inhalation. It does not allow for an accurate measurement because the inhalation phase starts prior to full exhalation and no flattening of the top of the measurement waveform. In other words, it is not end-tidal volume because the patient did not fully exhale before the next breath.

The curve below does show $P_{ET}CO_2$ > 45; however, we don't know how much greater it might have been if the patient had exhaled to end-tidal volume; because the next inhalation began so soon.

This waveform has no plateau, not accurate!

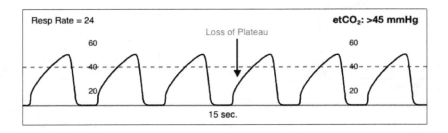

Illustration of capnograph waveform with an inaccurate reading

P_ECO_2 *Interpretation* –

Condition #1 - Waveform plateau is present and P_ECO_2 is displaying a number. This is accurate and reasonable to relate to P_aCO_2.

Condition #2 - Waveform plateau present and P_ECO_2 and correlates with P_aCO_2. Good for assessment of changes in the patient's minute volume and metabolism.

Condition #3 - Waveform plateau present and P_ECO_2 is much lower than P_aCO_2 Good for assessment of changes in deadspace to tidal volume ratio, V_D/V_T, and trending changes in minute volume and metabolism.

Condition #4 - Waveform **does not** plateau. Not accurate; marginal for trending minute volume and cannot be used for calculations. It is useful for crude monitoring of effectiveness of CPR and/or ET Tube placement. This would be similar to the less accurate, single-use carbon dioxide detection devices that merely indicate the presence of carbon dioxide or not. During CPR effective chest compressions produce cardiac output, and $ETCO_2$ will be present. Poor compressions or lack of cardiac output will soon result in zero $ETCO_2$. Placement of an endotracheal tube in the patient's esophagus will not show any carbon dioxide as opposed to the bronchi. These are measures of whether or not carbon dioxide is present at all.

Review: End-Tidal Carbon Dioxide ($ETCO_2$) measurement

1. Check for plateau on the waveform
2. Correlate with P_aCO_2 if possible
3. Always THINK about implications

ICU Nursing Monitor

The ICU nurse's monitor is a prominent device in the room usually located above the head of the bed to one side of the patient for easy access for the nurse to operate and respond to the monitor.

This is a physiologic monitor of many parameters including pulse, EKG strip, blood pressure, respiratory rate and pulse oximetry plus any number of other pressure monitors, carbon dioxide detector, along with a microprocessor to do special measurements and calculations.

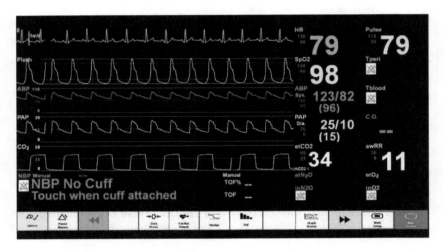

Illustration of the display screen of the ICU nurse's monitor

This monitor is a source of a great deal of information as well as a source of many audio and visual alarms of varying importance.

The ICU nurse's monitor transmits information to the ICU nursing station central monitor which is being visually monitored by ICU nurses, monitor technicians and/or the intensivist. The ICU nurse's patient monitor is also being electronically monitored by an ICU computer system that can automatically alarm and record events happening to the patient. This system is usually connected directly to the patient's electronic medical record system and has the ability to store data to retrieve for analysis of specific events or for printing for documentation.

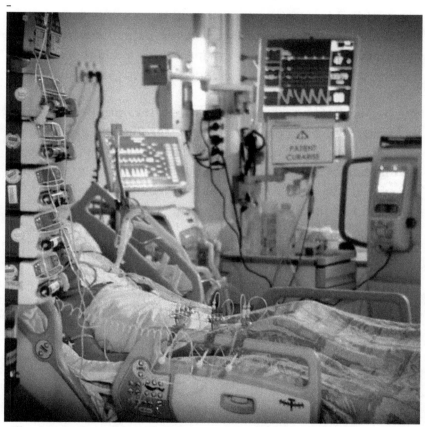

Illustration of an ICU patient with ventilator, ICU nurse monitor, IV pumps and other devices.

ICU Bed

The ICU bed is a sophisticated and expensive machine. It has to be mobile with large wheels to transport patients to special procedures and have places for multiple IV poles. Some have electric motors to propel them while in transit. An empty ICU bed can weigh up to 500 lbs.

The ICU bed has patient controls and nurse controls including the ability of the nurse to lock out the patient controls when necessary. It generally has the capacity for a 500 lb. patient. If patients are larger than 500 lbs., specialty beds are available.

The bed is electric and has microprocessor-controlled functions including taking the patient's weight, turning the patient from side to side by inflating and deflating portions of the mattress, having alarms set to alert the nurse if the patient is getting out of bed, the ability to raise and lower the entire bed or the head and feet independently. The bed can also be changed into a chair configuration. The whole bed can be tilted from flat to Trendelenberg which is a head down position.

During cardiopulmonary resuscitation (CPR) the bed has a CPR setting to provide a hard surface to improve chest compressions.

ICU beds are constructed with antimicrobial materials to facilitate cleaning. The headboard and footboard are easily removable to provide better access to the patient when necessary. An ICU bed can cost $60,000.

IV pumps

IV pumps are ubiquitous in ICU rooms. Patients will likely have multiple IV lines running several medications at the same time. There is no room for medication errors in ICU. These pumps are electronic and very precise. The IV pumps also have alarms set by the nurse for ease of medication delivery and patient safety.

Manual Resuscitator/ "Ambu"/Bag-valve Resuscitator

A self-inflating manual resuscitator is constantly present at the bedside of a patient on a ventilator. This device is usually connected to an oxygen flowmeter and can provide a high concentration of oxygen to the patient by connecting it to the endotracheal tube and squeezing the bag. If oxygen is not available, the resuscitation bag will self-inflate with room air after each breath. The single-patient use manual resuscitator is a very reliable piece of equipment with special attachments to provide PEEP similar to what the patient's ventilator is providing, and a simple pressure gauge to help keep from over pressuring the patient's lungs.

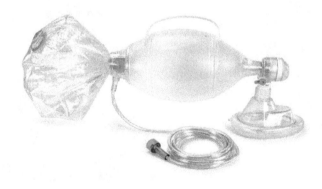

Illustration of manual resuscitator bag

Manual Resuscitator Bag Features

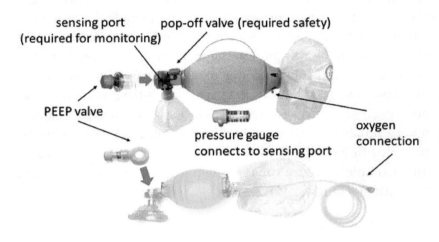

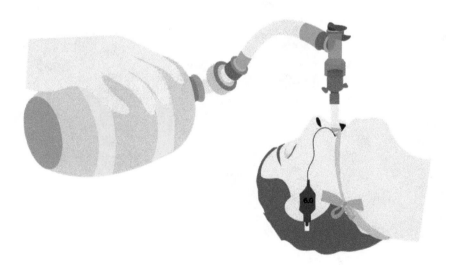

Illustration of a manual resuscitation bag in use

The manual resuscitator has about 1500 ml volume. When squeezed with one hand it can deliver up to 600 ml breath or tidal volume. It can deliver up to 1000 ml when squeezed with two hands. Please note these volumes are in excess of normal tidal volume. If the operator is excited in some emergency situation squeezing the bag fast and deeply, it is easy to hyperventilate the patient bringing their CO_2 down rapidly. It is also possible for the operator to get distracted and neglect to squeeze the bag. This seems unlikely but can easily happen when many things are happening at once during CPR, or during transport while exiting elevators, maneuvering narrow hallways, or dealing with other emergent problems.

Manual resuscitators have a built-in pressure relief valve set at 40 cmH_2O to protect the patient from overpressure injury (barotrauma). Fortunately, most operators are skillful and paying close attention, so this is not necessary. In emergencies some patients have such stiff lungs or obstructed airways that this high pressure is reached every breath.

If the patient needs to be breathed with a resuscitation bag for an extended period of time, it is wise to have a pulse oximeter and $ETCO_2$ measuring device attached.

For reasons described above, ventilator patients should not be transported between ICU and other areas using a manual resuscitator. Their ventilator should go with them or a similar specialized transport ventilator. This is a National safety standard that is sometimes bypassed for convenience, or because of arrogance of health care professionals who think manual resuscitators are as consistent as the ICU or transport ventilator.

Other equipment that may be present

There are a large number of machines that may be in an ICU patient's room that have nothing to do with the ventilator including dialysis machine, aortic balloon pump, DVT prevention compression device and others.

Initial Assessment: Does the Patient Need a Ventilator?

The patient/ventilator relationship is very complex. There are thousands of articles published in the medical literature, and scores of books have been written on the subject. In spite of the extensive study and published material there remains very little solid science in this endeavor; however, the more science can be interwoven into this relationship the more it seems to improve outcomes.

The complex relationship between the patient and the ventilator is managed in a number of ways and has several distinct phases, thus the organization of the following chapters of this book.

Chapter 4: **Assessment of the patient's condition** has to bring the medical team to the knowledge or belief that mechanical ventilation intervention is needed. This is often done in a matter of a few minutes or may be a well thought-out protocol that is implemented after days or weeks of planning. The patient's and/

or the family's wishes are an important factor in this decision-making process.

Chapter 5: **Initial mechanical ventilator settings** are established for the patient with a secure artificial airway. These settings will not only keep the patient alive, but will hopefully be close to physiologically normal or close to some predetermined goal.

Chapter 6: **Optimizing the patient/ventilator interface** may last a few minutes or as long as a few days. Here the healthcare team will try to support the patient's breathing with the greatest amount of comfort, least amount of interference and least number of complications.

Chapter 7: **Discontinuing mechanical ventilation** or getting the patient off the ventilator can be quick and easy or a prolonged miserable endeavor that ultimately fails.

Advanced Directives and Preferences (POLST)

Placing a patient on a ventilator is generally very anxiety producing. There is seldom a situation for mechanical ventilation without serious consequences. Anxiety for the patient, family and friends comes from the gravity of the situation. Anxiety for the healthcare team comes from the awesome responsibility of taking over one of the patient's most basic, important body functions and performing it artificially. Mechanical ventilation is an audacious action.

The assessment and decision to place a human being on a mechanical ventilator can be easy and straightforward or often extremely complex and difficult.

The following discussion is not properly legal or intended to give legal advice. The following discussion is to describe some legal documents and actions or inactions that influence whether or not a person might be supported by a mechanical ventilator. Hospitals can refer patients and families to proper legal advice.

Does the patient have "advanced directives" to clearly direct their end-of-life care? These are legal documents like Power of Attorney, "Living Will" or Last Will and Testament. Advanced Directives need to be made in advance with participation from the patient's physician, loved ones, and/or attorney as the patient wishes. If the patient has a known terminal disease and has legally documented their wishes to avoid resuscitative efforts and/or mechanical ventilation, they may choose not to get placed on mechanical ventilation nor receive other designated invasive or life support procedures. Each of these advanced directives documents are commonplace.

Very briefly, the Advanced Directive gives consent or refuses consent to any care, treatment, service, or procedure to maintain, diagnose, or otherwise affect a person's physical or mental condition. Advanced Directives may designate specific health-care providers and institutions, desire for organ donation; as well as address approval or disapproval of diagnostic tests, surgical procedures, use of mechanical ventilators, programs of medication, orders to resuscitate; and/or give artificial nutrition and hydration.

POLST (Physician Orders for Life-Sustaining Treatment) is an abbreviated type of Advanced Directive that states directly "Do or Do not Resuscitate" if the patient has no pulse or is not breathing. It can further specify if the person has a pulse and breathing that they may only want:

1. Comfort care, meaning pain relief and no advanced procedures.
2. Limited advanced interventions including choice of oxygen, endotracheal intubation, mechanical ventilation, bi-level positive pressure ventilation (NIV), and admission to ICU.
3. Full treatment; do everything.

The POLST needs to be signed and made readily available to Emergency Medical Services (Ambulance or Emergency Room) personnel. Emergency Medical Services (EMS) personnel will not search through a person's house for the POLST or advance directives. It is common practice to put the POLST on the refrigerator or some other obvious place. In addition, emergency medical services personnel are very unlikely to even read advance directives, because the document is too long and the legalese too complex in the face of a person dying in front of them. The POLST seems to be the best way to communicate with EMS personnel at this time.

If clear instructions are not available, the patient is given full treatment or "do everything." It is very difficult for a patient who is being resuscitated or has been intubated and is being mechanically ventilated to have those interventions reversed in the emergency room or immediately in the ICU. The legal implications are very complex and potentially costly.

Please see a POLST form below.

PROVIDER ORDERS FOR LIFE-SUSTAINING TREATMENT (POLST) - HAWAI'I

FIRST follow these orders. THEN contact the patient's provider. This Provider Order form is based on the person's current medical condition and wishes. Any section not completed implies full treatment for that section. Everyone shall be treated with dignity and respect.

Patient's Last Name

First/Middle Name

Date of Birth   Date Form Prepared

A
Check One

CARDIOPULMONARY RESUSCITATION (CPR): ** *Person has no pulse and is not breathing* **

☐ Attempt Resuscitation/CPR   ☐ Do Not Attempt Resuscitation/DNAR (Allow Natural Death)
(Section B: Full Treatment required)

If the patient has a pulse, then follow orders in **B** and **C**.

B
Check One

MEDICAL INTERVENTIONS: ** *Person has pulse and/or is breathing* **

☐ **Comfort Measures Only** Use medication by any route, positioning, wound care and other measures to relieve pain and suffering. Use oxygen, suction and manual treatment of airway obstruction as needed for comfort. *Transfer if comfort needs cannot be met in current location.*

☐ **Limited Additional Interventions** Includes care described above. Use medical treatment, antibiotics, and IV fluids as indicated. Do not intubate. May use less invasive airway support (e.g. continuous or bi-level positive airway pressure). *Transfer to hospital if indicated. Avoid intensive care.*

☐ **Full Treatment** Includes care described above. Use intubation, advanced airway interventions, mechanical ventilation, and defibrillation/cardioversion as indicated. *Transfer to hospital if indicated. Includes intensive care.*

Additional Orders: _____

C
Check One

ARTIFICIALLY ADMINISTERED NUTRITION: *Always offer food and liquid by mouth if feasible*
(See Directions on next page for information on nutrition & hydration)   *and desired.*

☐ No artificial nutrition by tube.   ☐ Defined trial period of artificial nutrition by tube.
                                                Goal:
☐ Long-term artificial nutrition by tube.

Additional Orders

D
Check One

SIGNATURES AND SUMMARY OF MEDICAL CONDITION - Discussed with:

☐ Patient or ☐ Legally Authorized Representative (LAR). If LAR is checked, you **must** check one of the boxes below:

☐ Guardian   ☐ Agent designated in Power of Attorney for Healthcare   ☐ Patient-designated surrogate

☐ Surrogate selected by consensus of interested persons (Sign section E)   ☐ Parent of a Minor

Signature of Provider (Physician/APRN licensed in the state of Hawai'i.)
My signature below indicates to the best of my knowledge that these orders are consistent with the person's medical condition and preferences.

Print Provider Name	Provider Phone Number	Date
Provider Signature (required)	Provider License #	

Signature of Patient or Legally Authorized Representative
My signature below indicates that these orders/resuscitative measures are consistent with my wishes or (if signed by LAR) the known wishes and/or in the best interests of the patient who is the subject of this form.

Signature (required)	Name (print)	Relationship (write "self" if patient)
Summary of Medical Condition	Official Use Only	

Unfortunately, many times these documents are either not available or used. For example, a terminally-ill patient with a well thought out "Do not resuscitate" plan collapses at home or quits breathing. A caregiver makes a panic call to 911. When the ambulance arrives if the legal documentation cannot be produced or is overlooked, or those present weren't "in the loop", or for many other reasons cannot go through with the patient's plan, the emergency medical services personnel of the ambulance and emergency department will go on protocol to do whatever is necessary to support the patient's life and body functions. Once a life is supported on a mechanical ventilator or a non-invasive ventilator it is much more complicated to get the patient off those machines. However, even at that point, it is possible and sometimes desirable to get the patient off sooner than later.

There is a sometimes-confusing issue with Advanced Directives in that they often contain the terminology of "in case of terminal illness" or "terminal disease or condition". The terminal status of a person or patient is determined by a physician. If the physicians involved do not think the patient is "terminal", life support and other aspects of advanced directives will be used to keep the patient alive. Sometimes this is to the surprise of the family, friends or even the patient. The physician has the knowledge and training to make this determination. In some rare cases disagreements about whether or not the patient is "terminal" end up in high profile court cases.

It is best to take care of this in advance, thus the term "Advanced Directives". It is best to communicate a person's wishes and preferences to significant caregivers, including appropriate family and friends.

If there are "Do not resuscitate" instructions and a person quits breathing or starts to die, significant others will want to call the person's primary care physician or hospice, not 911. Primary physicians or hospices will know what to do next without calling 911.

Patient History May Indicate Need for a Ventilator

The history of the patient is a very important piece of data: what is already known about the patient?

From where is the patient coming? Patients are most commonly assessed for the need for mechanical ventilation in the Emergency Room, Intensive Care Unit, Operating Room, or after respiratory failure during a stay on a hospital ward. Each area has a somewhat different set of variables to consider.

The Emergency Room has great variability in assessment for mechanical ventilation. For example, mechanical ventilation of an acute exacerbation of COPD will be much different than the type of ventilator intervention needed for a drug overdose, ARDS, pneumonia, multiple trauma from a motor vehicle crash, kidney failure, or a near-fatal asthma attack. Each of these problems must be addressed in a unique and individualized manner. Emergency room physicians must be appreciated as these assessments and terribly important decisions must be made accurately and quickly every time.

In the ICU these decisions are pretty straightforward as the patient has usually been in the medical center for a few hours or days. Most of these patients will have known multi-system failure, well-monitored vital signs, and an established rapport with the patient and significant others.

Operating Room variables must include the type of surgery. Mechanical ventilation of a neurosurgical patient may be much simpler and quite different from a patient recovering from heart surgery or lung surgery. It is usually known in advance if the surgical patient comes out of the operating room on a ventilator. Perhaps the patient simply needs ventilatory support until the anesthetic medications wear off.

The other areas of the medical center produce a wide spectrum of candidates for mechanical ventilation. These may be the survivors of cardiopulmonary failure and CPR efforts, patients who have become septic (infection in the blood), or respiratory decompensation from numerous other sources. This step up in care to the ICU and mechanical ventilation is often emergent.

The history of prior health problems is important. A patient with a history of COVD-19, pulmonary emphysema, acid/base disorders, neuromuscular weakness will be approached quite differently.

Physical Examination

Physical examination will be accomplished rapidly by several methods:

- Observation - Is the patient breathing? If yes, is it adequate? If not?
  - Is an artificial airway properly placed?
  - Is the airway secure?

- Is hand ventilation with bag/valve resuscitator adequate?
- What is the patient's appearance? Struggling? Blue? Responsive? Etc.
- What is the character of the secretions from the patient's airway?
  - Blood? Pus? Vomit?
- Auscultation – Listening with a stethoscope
  - Are breath sounds present over both lungs?
    - What is the quality of breath sounds? Wet? Bubbly? Wheezy? Too loud? Too soft? Absent?

Laboratory/X-ray Test Results

If there is time the physician will look at results from pulse oximetry and arterial blood gas tests. Arterial blood gases are great to assess adequacy of respiration showing clearly how much oxygen and carbon dioxide is in the blood. A chest x-ray can reveal a great deal about disorders in the lungs. We won't go deep into radiologic (x-ray) examination of the chest, because this topic deserves a book of its own.

Making the Decision to Ventilate, or Not

After considering the medical reasons to put a person on the ventilator, it is appropriate to consider, "Is this the right thing to do ethically?" This is a very difficult question at times. Technology has outstripped social development in this area. This is one point where this disparity comes to focus. If the patient and family were forward thinking, there would be some plan in place. Even with the plan in place, it often remains difficult because of the beliefs of specific physicians, family members or others. For example, a living will generally require that the patient have a terminal illness. This sounds easy, but it is not. One physician will determine that this particular respiratory failure is irreversible where another may not. Another example is where a physician may join the family at the bedside of a 90-year-old patient with metastatic cancer who is struggling to breathe and ask, "Do you want me to put a little tube in the mouth and relieve this struggling? How is the family to decline? A further example is when some family member knowing full well that the wishes of their parent or spouse is to not be placed on artificial mechanical ventilation will say, "Just do everything to keep them alive." It also happens that a family member who is assertive or aggressive convinces the others that a "miracle" is possible, and that they should disregard the patient's stated wishes, and/or the advice of a physician. Another frequent family request is "just keep him or her alive until" some loved one arrives from some distant place. Of course, this person in the distant place may not know of the situation or not have ready access to an airplane ticket. All of these situations and many more make this decision part of the initial assessment of the patient. It is also difficult for the physician to deny a loved one who is alive and well standing in front of them asking or demanding to prolong a patient's life in spite of the patient's stated directive not to be placed on a ventilator.

Alternatives to mechanical ventilation must be fully considered. This includes spontaneous breathing, death, non-invasive ventilation (NIV), and others.

Spontaneous breathing may be the option in the case of a patient who received just CPR at home, is successfully resuscitated and their cardiac problem treated. This patient will usually arrive at the Emergency Room being hand ventilated with a manual resuscitator. If the person doing the hand ventilation will slow down to a normal minute volume or slightly less than normal minute volume, often the patient will start breathing and maintain themselves quite well. If the operator of the manual resuscitator is overzealous and does not allow the patient's CO_2 to come back to normal, the patient may be placed on a ventilator unnecessarily.

Another alternative is sometimes painful as in our culture conversations about death and dying can be difficult. We tend to avoid the topic. When we talk about mechanical ventilator patients, death is unfortunately part of the conversation. If it is appropriate to the patient's disease process and wishes, sometimes it is best to allow them to die with dignity rather than prolonging their suffering for days or weeks in ICU on a ventilator.

Perhaps short term, non-invasive ventilation (NIV) with a face mask and "BiPAP" machine (Bi-level Positive Airway Pressure Ventilator) will support the patient and allow the medical team to reverse the breathing problem in a few hours. This will avoid the need for tracheal intubation and an ICU ventilator. The non-invasive ventilator and face mask will save the patient from the potential trauma of intubation and placement on an ICU ventilator. The decision to use NIV can easily transition into being put on an ICU ventilator if the underlying breathing problem cannot be resolved in a reasonable length of time. NIV should not be used for patients with Advanced Directives that forbid intubation and "mechanical ventilation"; because NIV, a "BiPAP" machine is a non-invasive "mechanical ventilator".

The bottom line with NIV/BiPAP is that it is a mechanical ventilator connected to the patient keeping them alive. It is often difficult to get the medical team to discontinue BiPAP because the patient will likely die according to their Advanced Directive and their wishes. At this point the patient may be intubated and put on an invasive mechanical ventilator. This is an awkward transition in modern medicine.

Side-effects, Complications and Dangers of Being on a Ventilator

Ventilator patients are extremely sick. So sick they will die if not placed on a ventilator. At the same time the ventilator supports the patient's life, it is exposing the patient to many possible side-effects, complications and dangers. Please see the list below.
When reading this list think of it as a list of nearly every possible, even rare, problems that could arise. It is a little like reading the warnings on a prescription drug information insert or signing a consent form for a surgical procedure. These are lists of most everything possible, and they range from common to very rare. It is important to remember that the ICU team is trying to reduce or prevent these problems constantly.

List of many side effects, complications, and dangers of being on a ventilator:

- Barotrauma
- Atelectrauma
- Volutrauma
- Pneumothorax
- Absorption atelectasis
- Oxygen toxicity
- Alveolar distention

- Aspiration
- Near-drowning
- ICU delirium, PTSD
- Hypercapnia/Hypercarbia
- Hyperventilation
- Hypoxemia
- Hypoxia
- Hypoventilation
- Hypocapnia/Hypocarbia
- Suffocation
- Pressure necrosis (oral, facial or tracheal)
- Vocal cord paralysis
- Trauma (due to intubation or suction)
- Infection
- Decreased blood pressure
- Reduced cerebral blood flow
- Fluid overload
- Decreased cardiac output
- Decreased renal function
- Tracheomalacia
- Tracheal stenosis
- Over sedation
- Death

If the reader is interested, a brief description of each follows in terms of how mechanical ventilation could possibly cause these problems.

Barotrauma - pulmonary barotrauma from invasive mechanical ventilation refers to alveolar rupture due to elevated pressure in the lungs. When the alveolar sac ruptures; air leaks into the area around the alveolus. When the air leaks out and around, it can result in conditions including pneumothorax

Volutrauma - lung injury caused by alveolar overdistension, overinflation

Atelectrauma - lung injury caused by high shear forces from repeated opening and collapse of atelectatic, but recruitable lung units.

VILI - ventilator-induced lung injury (VILI) can result in pulmonary edema, barotrauma, volutrauma, and worsening hypoxemia that can prolong mechanical ventilation, lead to multi-system organ dysfunction, and increased mortality.

PS-ILI - is generated by intense inspiratory effort yielding swings in transpulmonary pressure (i.e., lung stress); abnormal increases in transvascular pressure, producing pulmonary edema; an intra-lung shift of air between different lung zones; and/or diaphragmatic injury.

Pneumothorax - the presence of air or gas in the cavity between the lungs and the chest wall, causing collapse of the lung. This is caused by a hole in the lung letting air leak into the space just outside the lung, but inside the chest wall. The hole could be from high ventilator pressure or weak lungs or both.

Absorption atelectasis - Alveolar collapse secondary to the washout of nitrogen, an inert gas that normally helps maintain alveolar volume. Often ICU staff are tempted to increase the oxygen to 100% before and after tracheal suctioning in order to help the patient with any hypoxia caused by the suctioning procedure. This replaces the nitrogen in the alveolus with pure oxygen. If a particular alveolus is not ventilated well the oxygen may be all pulled out into the blood until the alveoli collapses like a deflated balloon. This collapse was caused by the absorption of all the oxygen with no nitrogen to hold the alveolus open.

Oxygen toxicity - exposure of the lungs to greater than 60% oxygen for periods exceeding 24-48 hours can lead to severe, irreversible pulmonary fibrosis.

Alveolar distention - overinflation of alveoli, very difficult to determine in real time.

Aspiration - inhalation of some foreign material; aspiration of vomitus, blood, or mucus may occur when a person is unconscious. When a person is conscious it usually causes choking. This can happen when fluid in the ventilator circuit is inadvertently dumped down the tracheal tube or when the tracheal tube cuff is deflated, and fluids pooled above the cuff pour into the lungs.

Near-drowning - is a term for those who survive the struggle against drowning. When a large amount of fluid is poured down into the lungs from the patient breathing circuit.

ICU delirium - an acute and fluctuating disturbance of consciousness and cognition, is a common manifestation of acute brain dysfunction in critically ill patients, occurring in up to 80% of the sickest intensive care unit (ICU) patients. ICU delirium can cause the patient to go "wild" and pull out critical tubes and inflict harm on themselves and others.

ICU Psychosis - Psychotic episode(s) occurring within 24 hours after entering the intensive care unit in patients with no previous history of psychosis; related to sleep deprivation, overstimulation, and time spent on life support systems.

PTSD - Post-traumatic stress disorder - a behavioral health condition that can develop after a person is exposed to a traumatic event, often life threatening. It is reported one in three ventilator survivors experience PTSD.

Hypercapnia/Hypercarbia - elevated carbon dioxide (CO_2) levels in the blood. Carbon dioxide is a product of the body's metabolism and is normally breathed out through the lungs. Caused by increased metabolism or decreased minute volume. Respiratory rate on the ventilator needs to be increased, if possible, to reverse this.

Hyperventilation - P_aCO_2 less than 35 - 45 mmHg. Does not mean breathing fast (tachypnea) or deeply (hyperpnea); although, that is what happens when normal people breath fast and deeply. Respiratory rate on the ventilator needs to be decreased, if possible. The patient might need to be sedated or have acidosis corrected by purposely reducing the P_aCO_2 to less than normal

Hypoxemia - low oxygen in the blood, P_aO_2 less than 80 - 100 mmHg, S_pO_2 less than 93 - 99%

Hypoxia - a general term describing less than normal amount of oxygen available to the body tissues

Hypoventilation - P_aCO_2 greater than 35 - 45 mmHg, Respiratory rate on the ventilator needs to be increased if possible, perhaps increase the tidal volume if it is too low.

Hypocapnia/Hypocarbia - lower than normal carbon dioxide (CO_2) levels in the blood. Carbon dioxide is a product of the body's metabolism and is normally breathed out through the lungs. Caused by decreased metabolism or increased minute volume, Respiratory rate on the ventilator needs to be decreased if possible. Patients may need to be sedated if the hypocapnia is caused by rapid, deep spontaneous breathing and they won't slow down.

Suffocation - stop or cut off breathing, caused by anything that interrupts the ventilator like kinked tubing, excessively long endotracheal suctioning, occlusion of ventilator tubing or ventilator failure.

Pressure necrosis (oral, facial or tracheal) - pressure against the skin caused by devices that secure the endotracheal tube to the lips or nose, or a face mask to the face in NIV, or pressure from the tracheal tube balloon against the wall of the trachea.

Vocal cord trauma/paralysis - the vocal cords are spread apart to place the endotracheal tube in the trachea. The vocal cords can be damaged during traumatic intubation, extubation and by abrasion by the endotracheal tube rubbing for days at a time.

Trauma (due to intubation or suction) - trauma to the delicate airways by placing endotracheal tubes, gastric tubes, and suction catheters.

Infection - ventilator patients have an increased risk of lung infection, central line infection, urinary tract infection and other hospital acquired infections.

Decreased blood pressure - positive pressure in the chest caused by ventilators can reduce the patient's blood pressure. This is difficult to sort out from other reasons, the blood pressure might drop, but in patients with blood pressure problems the interference by the ventilator increased pressures in the chest can be important

Reduced/increased cerebral blood flow - cerebral blood flow, and perfusion pressure can be changed by the positive pressure in the chest being transmitted to the brain as well as changes in carbon dioxide that can increase or decrease cerebral blood flows and pressures.

Fluid overload - ventilator patients generally have IVs providing nutrition (food and water) so it is easy to provide too much fluid, or the kidneys are failing, and fluid is building up in the body. This can cause pulmonary edema and lung problems.

Decreased cardiac output - ventilator positive pressure in the chest may decrease venous return to the right heart and decrease cardiac output causing fluid accumulation in the rest of the body.

Decreased renal function - if the cardiac output is decreased or the patient becomes severely hypoxic the kidneys can begin to fail.

Tracheomalacia - is abnormal softening of the cartilage of the trachea probably caused by irritation, lack of blood flow and stretching from the tracheal tube. The trachea is normally a rigid tube, but it can collapse with tracheomalacia.

Tracheal stenosis - is fibrotic and inflammatory changes the trachea probably caused by irritation, lack of blood flow and stretching from the tracheal tube. The trachea becomes narrowed and may present a problem breathing even long after the patient has come off the ventilator.

Over sedation - sedation is difficult to titrate and also depends on the patient's ability to metabolize the drugs; especially old people. If the patient is over sedated it will interfere with ventilator discontinuation/weaning.

Death - many people die on ventilators, but we hope it is from the underlying problem that caused respiratory failure not the life support ventilator. It does happen that some patients die from the side effects of the ventilator when high pressures and high oxygen levels are needed to keep the person alive. It is extremely rare that ventilators fail or catch on fire and kill ventilator patients.

The most powerful ventilator safety intervention is to get the patient off the ventilator! Reducing ventilator length of stay reduces risk of injury or death. Ventilator patients are probably at highest risk at ventilator initiation when the patient is being intubated and placed on initial settings. Another high-risk time is during intra-hospital transport where all sorts of unexpected occurrences might affect the patient's well-being.

Beyond that it is high risk all the time

Finally, a Decision is Made

After consideration of all this and more, the decision to place a person on a mechanical ventilator can be made.

CHAPTER 5

Placing the Patient on the Ventilator

Initial Settings: modes, rationales, standards of practice

A mechanical ventilator has many different variables that must be set appropriate to a specific patient. The first group is physician directed. These include:

Mode of ventilation	Ventilator controlled or patient controlled or some mix of both
Tidal Volume	6 – 12 ml/Kg.
Respiratory rate	6 – 20 breaths per minute
Oxygen (F_IO_2)	40– 100%
PEEP	5 – 10 Torr.
Pressure Support	5 – 10 cmH$_2$O

Mode of ventilation refers to whether the machine will let the patient take breaths of their own with the ventilator or whether the machine will initiate and define each breath. Mode of ventilation is a little more complex than this and can be broken down a couple of ways. Most simplistically there are two modes: Spontaneous mode and Mechanical mode.

Spontaneous mode - the ventilator allows the patient to start the breath, set a respiratory rate and breathe in as fast or slowly as they wish. For the most part the patient may take as deep a breath as they wish. However, the ventilator may be programmed to assist the patient to take a deeper breath, if necessary, by pushing in a little extra air.

Mechanical mode – the ventilator is programmed to provide the breath at set values like respiratory rate, tidal volume or peak pressure and flowrate and inspiratory time. Commonly, mechanical mode allows the patient to send a pressure or flow signal to trigger the ventilator when they want a ventilator breath.

Within mechanical mode there are fundamentally two ways of delivering the breath, Volume Control Ventilation (VCV) and Pressure Control Ventilation (PCV).

Volume Control Ventilation is a mode where the tidal volume of each mechanical breath is set on the ventilator, ex. 400 ml. Also the inspiratory flow rate and inspiratory time is set. The breath will be given to the patient at whatever pressure it takes to deliver that breath, within reasonable pressure limits.

Pressure Control Ventilation is a mode where the peak inspiratory pressure is set on the ventilator. Also the inspiratory time is set. The patient receives a variable tidal volume depending on how much air will go in over that time period at that amount of pressure, within reasonable pressure limits.

Within VCV and PCV are the modes most commonly ordered by physicians. Either PCV or VCV can be delivered by assist-control (AC) mode or Synchronized Intermittent Mandatory Ventilation (SIMV) mode.

AC mode is where all the variables defining a breath are programmed into the ventilator. The ventilator breathes the patient the same way every breath. AC allows the patient to signal the ventilator if they want a ventilator proscribed breath sooner than the set ventilator rate of breathing. The signal is when the patient starts a breath; a tiny pressure or flow change is sensed by the ventilator to give an "assist." So, the patient may breathe faster than the set rate with ventilator defined breaths or accept what the ventilator is programmed to deliver. The lowest respiratory rate acceptable for AC mode is 6 breaths/minute. If the patient is sedated and paralyzed, "medical coma", the ventilator will give breaths about 12 -15 times a minute while the patient does nothing. If the patient is fully awake, they get all the ventilator programmed breaths and any additional ventilator breaths they can signal the ventilator to give them.

SIMV mode is where spontaneous breathing is the primary mode of ventilation. It will be intermittently interrupted by the ventilator delivering a mechanical breath whenever the patient fails to initiate a spontaneous breath within a set time window. If the patient is initiating breathing at all, the intermittent mechanical breath is synchronized to the patient's inspiratory phase for comfort. If the patient is not breathing, "medical coma," the mechanical breaths take over just like AC mode. Respiratory rates for SIMV may be set as low as 1 breath every two minutes in a patient that is awake and strong enough to do most of the breathing.

APRV (Airway Pressure Relief Ventilation) mode is where the ventilator has a high pressure setting and a low pressure setting. The breath is held inside the patient's lungs at the high pressure setting for a set time and periodically released to the low pressure setting where it rushes out (exhales) for a set time, and then the ventilator pushes air into the lungs back to high pressure level (inhales). Meantime, between the set ventilator rate breaths the patient can breathe spontaneously at either the high or low pressure level. In APRV mode the patient will be controlled by the ventilator if they are in a medical coma, or they can do most of their own breathing if awake and strong enough.

Spontaneous mode is where the patient is allowed to breathe at their own respiratory rate and tidal volume. The ventilator supplies patient defined breaths. The patient has to be awake and strong enough to breathe. However, the patient may be assisted with each breath by an adjunct to ventilation called Pressure Support Ventilation (PSV).

PSV is sometimes called a mode of ventilation, but it is not. It is an additional pressure boost to spontaneous breaths in either "Spontaneous mode, SIMV, or APRV." It cannot be used with AC mode as there are no spontaneous breaths, only ventilator proscribed breaths. If this is confusing, don't worry it is confusing to a lot of people, even some medical professionals.

Automated modes of ventilation are found on a few ventilators. They are a mix of ventilator controlled and patient-controlled breaths with the microprocessor protocols embedded in the ventilator deciding what is best for the patient. The most sophisticated of these automated modes completely manage the patient's breathing whether in a medical coma or doing most of their own breathing. These modes will take the patient from complete ventilator dependency to ventilator discontinuation without health care practitioner interference. Automated ventilation can be more safe, comfortable and intelligent in managing the patient than non-automated modes.

Although these automated modes are called modes, actually they are not modes, but ventilator management protocols embedded in the ventilator's microprocessor. The ventilator is allowed to choose from a number of modes described above and manage the patient. Some of these automated ventilators can successfully manage the sickest ARDS patients. Automated ventilation modes have proprietary names such as Adaptive Support Ventilation (ASV) Hamilton Medical, Adaptive Ventilation Mode (AVM) Vyaire, SmartCare/PS Draeger, and Neurally Adjusted Ventilatory Assist (NAVA), Marquet, plus others. There is a great deal of experience and research published on these automated modes, so they are not experimental. This should become the future of mechanical ventilators.

There are also many hybrid modes of ventilation that combine limited automation on ventilators to optimize various aspects of the delivered breath. These usually have proprietary names like Proportional Assist ventilation (PAV+), Covidien, AVAPS, VAPS, etc. It is quite an alphabet soup, and it would be wise to ask the respiratory therapist to explain how a particular hybrid mode works.

Most often the physician will order the patient to be on some form of SIMV or AC mode using VCV with its set tidal volume, or PCV with its set pressure.

Tidal volume is the size of the normal breath. Tidal volume is measured and discussed in milliliters or decimal fractions of a liter. (See the illustration in Chapter 2) Physicians usually order tidal volumes between 5 – 12 ml/Kg body weight. Ideal body weight used in these calculations is taken from ideal body weight charts or from the physician's experience. There is a rationale for larger tidal volumes (12 – 15 ml/Kg) to keep the lungs open and prevent lung collapse, but it is not used so often. More recently low tidal volumes (4 – 8 ml/Kg) have become popular with research showing better outcomes for ARDS patients in AC mode. This may not be generalized to other types of patients or other modes of ventilation, since the most extensive research on size of tidal volume has been done on ARDS and AC mode. Some practitioners have generalized the protocol to all disease entities and other modes of ventilation.

Respiratory rate or "frequency" is the number of breaths per minute. Respiratory rate will be initiated between 6 – 20 breaths/minute. Physicians will generally order a frequency that will provide adequate minute volume without overtaxing the patient's ability to breathe spontaneously. More specifically the physician will want the P_aCO_2 between 35 – 45 mmHg. to keep the patient's pH between 7.35 - 7.45. There should be a clear reason for starting outside this P_aCO_2 and pH range. Whenever the patient's $P_aCO_2 > 45$ mmHg, generally the ventilator rate will be increased to "blow off" CO_2 back to normal range. When the patient's $P_aCO_2 < 35$ mmHg. the ventilator rate will be decreased to help the patient retain CO_2. These adjustments are not just a formality as the P_aCO_2 is a primary acid (carbonic acid) for regulating the patient's acid- base balance in their blood, brain and body. An artificially elevated or lowered P_aCO_2 should be a planned maneuver, not something done by default or by not paying attention to patient assessment. We will discuss rationale for purposely altering the patient's acid-base balance via P_aCO_2 adjustment by setting high or low respiratory rates later in this chapter. Often the physician will initially order a respiratory rate that will take all the work of breathing from the patient until the causes of respiratory failure or the reasons for mechanical ventilation can be further assessed.

Positive End Expiratory Pressure (PEEP) of 5 - 10 mmHg. is the amount of pressure held in the patient's lungs at the end of exhalation. PEEP can be considered a baseline pressure being held in the patient's lungs. In the diagram below the horizontal line is zero pressure. The blue line is the patient's pressure tracing. The PEEP is an increased pressure baseline holding pressure inside the lungs at all times.

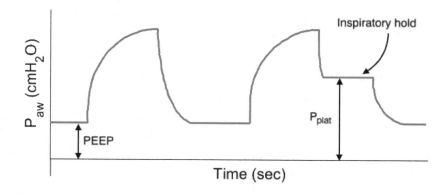

PEEP of 5 - 10 cmH$_2$O is a common initial setting. It is believed that bypassing structures in the upper airway with an endotracheal tube causes a person to lose Functional Residual Capacity (FRC). FRC is the normal amount of air remaining in our lungs at the end of a normal quiet exhalation. PEEP is associated with an increase in air trapped in the lungs or FRC. PEEP is used to keep the lungs "open" in the cases where lung diseases cause collapse of the airways and alveoli. PEEP use in this manner might be the only function of a ventilator that is actually therapeutic (helps them get better) versus supportive (just keeps them alive).

Oxygen Concentration (F_IO_2) of 40 -60% where F is

Fraction, I is Inspired, and O_2 is Oxygen, or percentage of oxygen in the air the ventilator is providing the patient. It is properly expressed as a decimal fraction but is most commonly referred to as a percentage. Oxygen is initially set between 40% - 100%. Over the short term, minutes to an hour, oxygen is not toxic. Lack of oxygen can be damaging or fatal. With that in mind the physician will generally start a patient on 100% oxygen unless there is data available to show that a lower F_IO_2 is safe. This data is often available from prior pulse oximetry or arterial blood gas analysis. It is important to remember that atmospheric air is 21% oxygen, and that oxygen <40 - 60% is considered by many to be non-toxic for relatively long periods of time.

Pressure Support of 5 - 10 cmH_2O is an initial setting

for any patient that is breathing spontaneously or is in a mode that allows spontaneous breaths. Pressure support almost literally gives the patient a pressure boost during the inspiratory phase. The idea behind using some pressure support on any spontaneously breathing patient is that the ventilator, breathing circuit, and artificial airway cause an imposed work of breathing or inspiratory resistance to breathing that is higher than normal. For most ventilator patients this is about $8 - 10$ cmH_2O. Some systems might be considerably higher. Additionally, the physician may choose to use higher levels of pressure support to relieve the patient from work of breathing and help them achieve a larger tidal volume during a spontaneous breath. Excellent ventilators measure and report inspiratory resistance, so the practitioner can better adjust the pressure support.

The remainder of the ventilator settings are numerous and are set by the respiratory therapist. These settings are mainly to match the ventilator to the patient for comfort and setting of alarms for safety. They include:

Sensitivity	flow sensitivity or flow trigger = 1 – 5 L/min or pressure sensitivity or pressure trigger = -1 – -3 cmH$_2$O
Waveform	descending ramp
Peak flow	30 – 60 L/min.
Inspiratory temp.	37 degrees C. (98.6 F.) and 100% relative humidity at the airway
Sigh	not needed
Rise time	50 msec.
ETS	25%
Alarm Settings	as appropriate, guidelines below

Let's look at each parameter.

Sensitivity is the way the patient communicates to the ventilator that they want a breath right now. The ventilator is either watching for a slight pressure drop caused by the patient trying to suck a breath in through the closed system or a slight generation of inspiratory flow in the opposite direction of the exhalation. The less effort the patient has to exert, the more sensitive the ventilator. Sensitivity setting is sometimes called "trigger." It is the patient's trigger for getting the machine to shoot out a breath.

During patient-initiated breaths the trigger is a drop in airway pressure or inspiratory flow generated by the patient starting to take a breath. This change is "sensed" by the ventilator and the ventilator responds by initiating a breath in less than 100 milliseconds in some ventilators. All ventilators are pretty fast, so the patient can be reasonably comfortable.

From the patient's bedside you should be able to determine if the patient is triggering the ventilator by looking for an indicator light that comes on briefly each time the patient takes a breath. The indicator may be labeled "Trigger" or "Auto." This is an important observation because you can tell if the patient has respiratory drive or is unable to even start to take a breath. Also, if the patient looks like they are trying to breathe and the trigger indicator is not coming on, perhaps the ventilator/patient interface needs adjustment.

The most sensitive trigger is a proprietary product on the Maquet, Servo ventilator called Neurally Adjusted Ventilatory Assist (NAVA). This works with a sensor placed down the patient's throat deep in the esophagus near the diaphragm. It senses the neurally transmitted electrical signal sent by the brain. NAVA is probably the best sensitivity available; it is just limited to one brand of ventilator and requires an extra sensor placed inside the patient's esophagus.

Flow trigger is the microprocessor-based ventilator provides a base flow through the breathing circuit. The ventilator "watches" the in-flow and out-flow; whenever differences are detected the ventilator is triggered to provide a breath. The response time of this system is critical.

Sensitivity is set to allow the patient to most comfortably initiate spontaneous or mechanical breaths without confusing the ventilator. If the sensitivity is set too low the ventilator will "auto-cycle" or chatter off and on, which is very uncomfortable to the patient. If the sensitivity is set too high, it will be too hard for the patient to trigger a breath.

If the patient does not initiate a breath, the default trigger is time. After a certain time has elapsed, usually a few seconds, the ventilator will give a mechanical breath.

In the ventilator monitor tracing below, the green line is flowrate vs. time. When the green line goes above zero is inspiration (air flowing into the patient). When the green line is below zero, it is exhalation (air flowing out of the patient). You can see in the close-up box that if the patient starts to suck in a little air, the ventilator follows immediately with a breath.

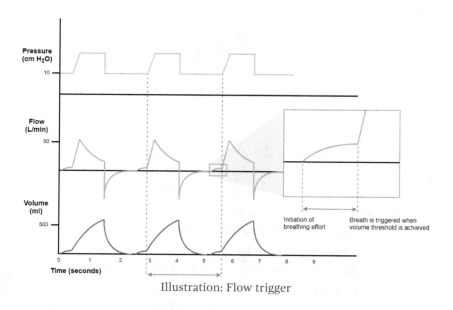

Illustration: Flow trigger

Pressure trigger – at the beginning of inspiration the patient is pulling against a closed system and causes a slight pressure drop in the patient's chest, airways and ventilator circuit. A simple pneumatic or electronic feedback triggers the ventilator to provide a breath. The response time of this system is critical. In the graph below you can see the yellow line dip slightly for a very short time to "normal trigger." If the patient does not initiate a breath to trigger the machine, the machine will automatically trigger when it is time for the next ventilator breath.

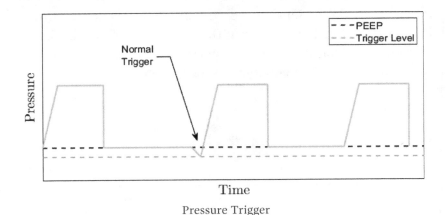

Pressure Trigger

Waveform refers to the shape of the inspiratory flow rate graphed against time. The square wave is the simplest wave form to imagine. If the ventilator rapidly opens a valve to a set flowrate, e.g. 40L/min., allows the gas to flow constantly at that rate during the breath, and rapidly shuts the valve at the end of inhalation. This would be the rectangular or square waveform. Since the inspiratory valves of the ventilator have very rapid response time and very precise control of gas flow the microprocessor can be programmed to deliver a number of different flow waveforms. Most ventilators have a choice of two or more waveforms.

Flow Curves

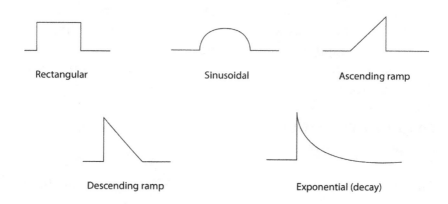

| Rectangular | Sinusoidal | Ascending ramp |

| Descending ramp | Exponential (decay) |

The descending ramp has been shown to have some advantages over the other waveforms. So, it is a good place to start.

Peak flow - the highest flow rate reached during any part of the inspiratory phase. This would be the highest peak on the inspiratory flow waveforms above.

Normal resting peak flow is about 30 L/min. Normal maximal effort peak flowrate is between 300 – 600 L/min. Initial ventilator settings are usually 50 – 60 L/min.

Inspiratory time - the time in seconds for the inspiratory phase of the respiratory cycle. The initial setting is between 0.5 and 2.0 secs. depending on the respiratory rate. Inspiratory time is not usually set during VCV as the tidal volume, peak flow and respiratory rate define the inspiratory time. Inspiratory time is a necessary adjustment during PCV.

Peak flow, tidal volume, inspiratory time, Inspiratory:Expiratory ratio (I:E ratio), and respiratory rate all interact depending on the type of ventilator, mode of ventilation and what is being changed. As a result, one or more of these parameters may default to what is required for a primary choice of setting. Example, if we turn the respiratory rate setting down the inspiratory time might have to be shorter, or if we increase the I:E ratio setting the inspiratory time may need to be longer.

Inspiratory temperature – inspired gas temperature at the patient's airway

This is initially set at 37 degrees C. (98.6 degrees F.) and 100% relative humidity.

It is important to humidify and warm the inspired gas because the artificial airways by-pass the patient's normal mechanisms for warming, humidifying and filtering inspired air. The normal mechanisms are the nose and mucus membranes of the upper airways.

This can be accomplished with a heated humidifier or HME (heat/moisture exchanger). An HME is a small device located in the ventilator circuit that acts like an artificial nose.

HME is adequate in most cases but has limitations. Limitations to the HME are when the inspiratory flowrate is beyond the specifications of the HME or when the patient is coughing up large amounts of mucoid or bloody secretions. The secretions may shoot out of the patient's airway during exhalation and plug up the HME.

Sigh – periodic hyperinflation of the lungs. This function was added to ventilators in the early 1970s when patients were not able to breath spontaneously with the ventilator. Every breath was a mechanical breath of the same size and description. It was thought that a person might periodically need a deeper breath. These "sighs" might be set at 1.5 or 2 times the tidal volume and would be set to occur several times an hour. Now that smaller tidal volumes are more popular again periodic sigh may be used more often.

Rise time (P$_{ramp}$) – the set amount of time the ventilator is allowed from the beginning of inspiration to reach PSV and/or PCV pressure level. Rise time is how fast the ventilator accelerates the flowrate to reach some pressure goal. Sometimes it is called "Pressure ramp". In the diagram below are three different rise times, each one a little longer than the previous one. Let's say 50, 100 and 150 millisecs.

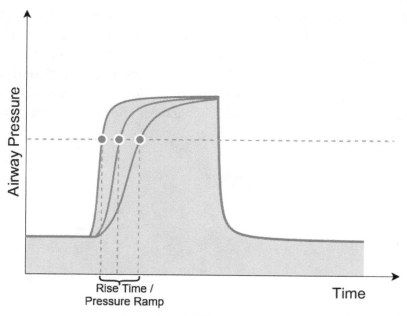

Illustration: 3 different rise times

Rise time of 50 millisecs (msec) is a reasonable initial setting. Some ventilators are programmed at this rise time, and it is not adjustable. It may be increased to as much as 200 msec. as needed.

Setting rise time can help better match the patient to the ventilator. If the patient has a rapid or gasping inspiration, a shorter rise time seems more comfortable. The short rise time allows them to get a higher initial flow rate to meet their needs. If the patient is breathing very slowly, a longer rise time may be more comfortable. The short rise time seems to almost surprise such a patient with excessive flow.

Expiratory Trigger Sensitivity (ETS) is the criteria

that terminates expiratory phase in spontaneous breathing with pressure support ventilation. It is also called expiratory flow trigger. In other words, after the patient has taken a breath of their own and the ventilator has given them a boost with increased pressure, they start to exhale. During that exhalation the ventilator computer is looking at the flowrate of the air coming out of the patient. When the flowrate of the air coming out drops to, let's say 25% of the peak flow of the inspiratory phase, the ventilator will end exhalation and initiate the next breath.

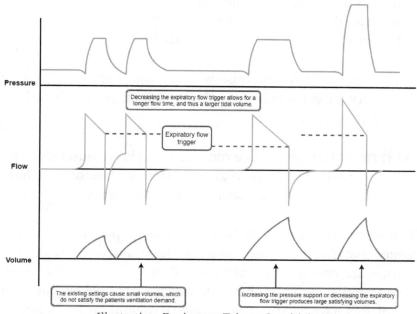

Illustration: Expiratory Trigger Sensitivity

The criteria are either a percentage of the peak flow or a set flow rate. When the manufacturer sets these, they are often 25% of peak flow or 10 L/min. Some ventilators are programmed at this expiratory trigger, and it is not adjustable. Newer devices allow the user or microprocessor to vary these settings. ETS = 25% is a good initial setting. The range of ETS adjustment is 10 to 40% of peak flow during the spontaneous breath.

You can see in the green flow curve above. The first expiratory flow trigger might be about 50% of peak flow where the second might be about 15 or 20% of the peak flow.

Setting ETS can help match the patient to the ventilator. If the patient is breathing rapidly, a shorter ETS, higher percentage, will keep them more comfortable. This allows the patient to complete a breath sooner and get on with the next breath. If the patient is breathing slowly and the spontaneous tidal volume is lower than desirable, a long ETS, lower percentage or flow rate, will allow the patient more time to exhale.

A good respiratory therapist will be adjusting rise time and expiratory trigger sensitivity to keep a spontaneously breathing patient more comfortable.

Alarm Settings – numerous physiologic measurements are being monitored by the ventilator at all times. Many of them have associated audio alarms, visual alarms and/or back-up systems.

Ventilator alarms need to be set at values that assure patient safety and do not cause needless noise and confusion. The alarms are covered in greater detail in Chapter 3. Machines. Some ventilators do not have each alarm listed below, but most ventilators have most of them. Note Hi pressure is listed first as it is most important.

Usual initial settings are:

Pressure	Hi	10 cmH$_2$O above peak inspiratory pressure
	Lo	5 cmH$_2$O above PEEP and below pressure support level
Tidal volume	Hi	50 – 100 ml above the largest, frequent tidal volume
	Lo	100 ml above calculated anatomic deadspace (2.2 ml/KG of body weight or 1.0 ml/lb. body weight)
PEEP	Hi	10 cmH$_2$O above set PEEP
	Lo	5 cmH$_2$O below set PEEP

Minute volume	Hi	1.0 liter above minute volume goal
	Lo	1.0 liter below minute volume goal
F_IO_2 (Oxygen %)	Hi	5% above F_IO_2 setting
	Lo	5% below F_IO_2 setting
Temp	Hi	2 degrees above temperature goal (37 degrees C.)
	Lo	2 degrees below temperature goal (37 degrees C.)
Apnea time		20 secs.
Apnea Backup		This is quite specific to the type of ventilator. Sometimes respiratory rate and tidal volume are chosen by operator or programmed by design engineers.

Place the ventilator on the patient

After the initial settings have been made and the ventilator placed on the patient, the patient must be assessed immediately.

First Patient/Ventilator Assessment:

Observation: Is there chest excursion? (Is the chest and/or abdomen going up and down). This sounds too simple but is absolutely important.

(Visual)

Is mechanical ventilation adequate? (Is the patient's color good and not struggling)

Appearance of the patient (Patient looks reasonably comfortable, all things considered)

Appearance of the ventilator (Have the lights and "sirens" turned off and quiet)

Auscultation: Presence of breath sounds bilaterally with a stethoscope (must place the stethoscope on each side of the chest to be certain both lungs are ventilating)

Quality of breath sounds (reasonable sounding gas flow in and out of the lungs)

Assess the patient/ventilator relationship immediately by measuring and documenting ventilation parameters including exhaled tidal volume, peak airway pressure, respiratory rate, minute volume, level of PEEP, mean airway pressure (MAP), plateau pressure, resistance, compliance, inspiratory time (T_I), expiratory time (T_E), I:E ratio, oxygen saturation by pulse oximetry (S_pO_2), and end-tidal carbon dioxide (P_ECO_2).

At the same time hemodynamic factors should be documented including blood pressure, heart rate and central venous pressure (CVP). Pulmonary artery pressure (PAP), pulmonary artery occlusion pressure (PAOP), and cardiac output (Q) should be measured and documented if a pulmonary artery (Swan-Ganz) catheter is in place. This is necessary because the heart and lungs share the same space, i.e. inside the chest. The way we manage the ventilator can affect cardiac function.

Next the ventilator settings must be documented, so a baseline relationship between the measured physiologic factors above and the ventilator settings can be established. This will usually include mode, tidal volume, peak airway pressure, respiratory rate, minute volume, PEEP, T_I, T_E, I:E ratio, sensitivity, pressure support.

At this time the respiratory therapist documents endotracheal tube placement including tube size, its position relative to the teeth or external nare (nostril), and endotracheal tube cuff (balloon) pressure. This is necessary because the patency of the airway (being unobstructed) is essential to the use of the ventilator. When the patient is moving, salivating and perhaps chewing and biting the endotracheal tube, it can move slowly or rapidly out of place and occasionally cause a brief disaster. It must be monitored closely. In addition, results of a post-endotracheal intubation chest x-ray should be documented to assure the proper placement of the ET tube.

After being assured that the patient is safe and heading in a reasonable direction while being supported by the ventilator, the patient will need to be allowed some time to equilibrate to this new level of ventilatory support and oxygenation. Immediate feedback from the pulse oximeter and $ETCO_2$ detector is very helpful.

After about 30 minutes an arterial blood gas sample is taken to assess the outcomes of the initial settings. The healthcare staff should be sure to correlate S_PO_2 and P_ECO_2 with P_aO_2, and P_aCO_2 respectively. It is a good time to calculate deadspace ventilation (V_D/V_T), right-to-left intrapulmonary shunt fraction (Q_S/Q_T) and calibrate the S_vO_2 monitor on the oximetric Swan-Ganz catheter if one is in place.

If this all seems very confusing and complicated, it is. It is a good time for the patient's loved ones to observe the new configuration and ask questions.

CHAPTER 6

Optimizing the Patient/ Ventilator Relationship

Now the patient has just been placed on the ventilator and has begun to stabilize.

We have to ask ourselves again, "Why is this patient on a ventilator?" We must have a clear answer and a plan to resolve that problem and get the person off the ventilator.

We have to ask ourselves every day, every shift and every visit, "Why is this patient on a ventilator?"

Anytime we can safely reduce the invasiveness of the ventilator, we must. Most invasive is oxygen over 40%, PEEP over 8 cmH_2O, and removal of the patient's ability to breathe on their own.

At the same time, we have to ask ourselves, "Are we doing everything possible to keep this patient safe? Being on a ventilator is much riskier than flying in an airplane. We must make every effort to eliminate errors. The ventilator patient is exposed to so much risk not being able to breathe, being dependent on a machine and healthcare providers for life support.

We also want to focus on the patient's comfort and find ways to help them tolerate an almost intolerable situation. Keeping the ventilator as comfortable as possible and reducing unnecessary alarms is helpful.

Matching the Ventilator to the Patient

The scenario is that we have now allowed time for the patient/ventilator relationship to equilibrate and have received results of our first assessments of this situation. An alternative scenario is that the patient/ventilator relationship is constantly changing, and we are at any point of maintaining the patient on artificial ventilation. Here the healthcare team will try to support the patient's breathing with the greatest amount of comfort, least amount of interference and least amount of complications. More specifically, the least amount of pressure, volume, mechanical breaths, and oxygen necessary to support the patient without overtaxing the patient's condition will be used. This may mean that the ventilator does all the breathing at high pressures and high F_IO_2, or it may mean that the ventilator supplies minimal pressure support to a spontaneous breathing patient on a low F_IO_2.

The physician will direct the changing of mode of ventilation, tidal volume, respiratory rate, F_IO_2 and PEEP either by direct order or via pre-approved protocol. Other ventilator settings or adjustments fine tuning the patient/ventilator will be changed by the respiratory care practitioner. All changes will be documented in the patient's record.

Review: Why do patients need a ventilator?

1. Lung/Thoracic Compliance Decreased: Their lungs or chest wall are too stiff, leathery or fibrous.
2. Airway Resistance Increased: Their breathing tubes (bronchial tubes) are obstructed, too narrow or blocked.
3. Impaired Neural Control of Breathing: breathing muscles are not getting a signal from the brain to breathe.
4. Weak Muscles of Respiration: breathing muscles are too weak to get enough breath.
5. R-L Intrapulmonary Shunt Increased: blood going to their lungs is not finding aerated alveoli.
6. Deadspace ventilation: increased: air coming into the lungs is not finding blood supply to alveoli.

The doctor may know in advance that this person will have respiratory failure. Then they are put on a ventilator before they experience respiratory failure.

These reduce down to basically two problems:

Ventilatory failure   primary assessment is P_aCO_2 – adjust by changing respiratory rate

Oxygenation failure   primary assessment is P_aO_2 – adjust by changing F_IO_2 or PEEP

Ventilatory Failure, what to do about it?

The patient in ventilatory failure is unable to ventilate, move enough air in and out of the lungs, to remove carbon dioxide from the body. A mechanical ventilator can ventilate patients, in almost all cases, enough to remove excess P_aCO_2. Minute volume and metabolic activity contribute to P_aCO_2 level in the blood. Arterial blood gas analysis is used to assess P_aCO_2.

If the arterial blood gas results assessing the initial settings has a P_aCO_2 outside normal limits (35 – 45 Torr.), we will change the minute volume of the ventilator accordingly by adjusting the respiratory rate. Respiratory rate will be increased, so the patient will ventilate more, and this change will lower the P_aCO_2. The respiratory rate will be decreased to raise the P_aCO_2, so the patient will ventilate less. The most common problem by far is too much P_aCO_2.

Changing tidal volume will also change P_aCO_2. For example, increasing the tidal volume will ventilate the patient more and reduce P_aCO_2. Why is respiratory rate chosen to change P_aCO_2? Generally, the tidal volume has been chosen according to one of the philosophies described above in the section on initial settings. Since the tidal volume setting is protecting the lung or opening the lung at its specific volume, it is more convenient to change the respiratory rate. If the patient is in PCV mode, P_aCO_2 can be also changed by increasing the peak pressure or lowering the PEEP. Once again, the rationale for choosing peak pressure of PCV or choosing PEEP level makes it more convenient to change the respiratory rate in PCV.

If the patient cannot be brought into P_aCO_2 range of 35 – 45 mmHg., at a respiratory rate of < 25 – 30 breaths per minute, physicians will usually begin trying other methods of increasing ventilation. This may include increasing tidal volume, changing mode of ventilation. The respiratory therapist may try changing inspiratory waveform, peak flow rate, I:E ratio, rise time or any other ventilator adjustment that might allow the patient to improve ventilation.

It is important to note the human bodies' acid-base balance is tied to P_aCO_2. Carbon dioxide carried in the blood ends up dissolved in the blood plasma as carbonic acid. Carbonic acid is a very dynamic factor in maintaining adequate acid-base balance in the blood; therefore, if the P_aCO_2 goes up, we get more carbonic acid in the blood and the blood becomes more acidic. If the P_aCO_2 goes down, we get less carbonic acid in the blood and the blood becomes more basic.

Ventilator management includes watching the blood pH and responding accordingly to big changes in the P_aCO_2.

If the inadequate ventilation persists in spite of this, and the peak inspiratory pressure approaches dangerous levels of 50 – 60 mmHg. Now the patient is in a very difficult situation and any number of less usual strategies may be pursued.

It is important to remember that in certain types of patients, maintenance of P_aCO_2 outside normal limits is desirable.

a. Some COPD (pulmonary emphysema, chronic bronchitis) patients require a P_aCO_2 of 50 – 60 mmHg. or greater, as they have chronic ventilatory failure. Their body has adjusted to a higher P_aCO_2 than normal.
b. Patients with a severe, acute metabolic acidosis will be managed with P_aCO_2 < 25 mmHg. in order to bring the pH toward normal (Generally, abnormally low pH is more harmful for a patient than low P_aCO_2).
c. Patients with head trauma either from surgery or injury are often managed with P_aCO_2 < 25 mmHg. (Carbon dioxide is a cerebral vasodilator, causing the blood vessels to the brain to open up). Reducing P_aCO_2 can constrict arteries to the head and reduce intracranial pressure temporarily.)

d. There is a concept called "Permissive hypercapnia". This concept is evoked whenever the healthcare team fails to be able adequately to ventilate the patient within "acceptable" limits. Rather than harm the patient with excessive pressures or volumes to reduce the P_aCO_2, the physician will decide that letting the P_aCO_2 build-up >45 mmHg. is a less dangerous alternative. The upper limit of permissive hypercapnia has not been established. Permissive hypercapnia is more often used with ARDS patients.

The ICU team must first identify the ventilatory problem and reverse the underlying cause of this ventilatory failure

Ventilatory Failure Problem #1 - Decreased lung compliance

Decreased lung compliance is loss of elasticity of the lung tissue or chest wall. When the lung and chest wall become less elastic it becomes more difficult for the muscles of inspiration to suck air into the lungs. This results in increased P_aCO_2. Lung compliance can get so low that the respiratory muscles will fail to ventilate adequately no matter how hard they work. The person will experience ventilatory failure and subsequent death unless the problem is reversed, or they are placed on mechanical ventilation which gives time for the problem to be reversed. A most concerning cause of decreased lung compliance is disruption of the alveolo-capillary membrane by any event that causes thickening, flooding, inflammation, or collapse. This is one of the primary problems in ARDS. ARDS causes the lung to be stiff, and heavy and decreases compliance. The cause of

ARDS must be identified, treated and the patient kept alive with mechanical ventilation until the treatment works and the patient's lung has healed. COVID-19 causes some sort of ARDS. PEEP is one of the few ventilator parameters that can be therapeutic. If PEEP can be used to hold the lung open to a point where the compliance is better, the patient can be ventilated at this baseline pressure and allow for larger tidal volumes to be used at lower peak pressures. Within reasonable limits this can help protect the lung from too much volume or pressure and in the end when the patient is well enough to start breathing spontaneously, it can help make their efforts more effective. To understand this better, think of blowing up a new balloon. It is hard to get the balloon to open initially, decreased balloon compliance. Then it becomes easier to blow up as the balloon's compliance drops at larger volumes. If we were letting air in and out of a balloon, it might be a good trick to not let it go completely flat each time. We think this is why we use PEEP.

Ventilatory Failure Problem #2 - Increased Airway Resistance

Airway resistance refers to the amount of pressure it takes to move air through the bronchial tubes or occasionally other structures in the patient's airway including the trachea, larynx, pharynx, nose, mouth and any artificial airways that have been used to connect the ventilator. The easiest way to understand this problem is to breathe through a paper towel tube, a large drinking straw, a standard size drinking straw and a small coffee stirring straw.
Each time the radius of the airway is cut in half it becomes 16 times harder to breathe through the tube.

The more common reasons that a patient's airways are narrowed include inflammation (swelling closed) like asthma or bronchitis, occlusion of the airway with thick mucus, an inhaled foreign object, a tumor, or constriction of the airway tube by muscle contraction around the outside wall (asthma) or scarring from irritation or surgery.

The cause of airway narrowing which is causing the resistance to air movement must be identified and reversed. A ventilator may be required while this is being done.

Ventilatory Failure Problem #3 - No Signal to Breathe

The breathing regulatory system in the brain and the conducting nerves can be interrupted in a number of ways. Sedative drug overdose or "medical coma" where sedatives, paralytic and/ or other drugs put the breathing centers to sleep or block the nerves from the brain to the respiratory muscles. This can usually be easily reversed if a ventilator keeps the person alive during the process. Strokes (blood clots to the brain) cerebral vascular bleeding like cerebral aneurysms rupturing can block the respiratory centers. Of course, various types of trauma or suffocation can cause varying degrees of damage to the breathing centers in the brain. In these cases, reversing the problem may work, and it may not. Either way a ventilator may be needed until the problem is assessed, treated, becomes well or the patient is determined to be terminal or brain dead. It is also possible for the nerves from the head to the diaphragm to be damaged during trauma like a broken neck or cut during surgery. Without the diaphragm working the patient will need mechanical ventilation until some other solution can be implemented.

Ventilatory Failure Problem #4 - Weak Breathing Muscles

Breathing muscles do not tire out during normal breathing unless something else is wrong. Muscle weakness diseases are not that common, but can be devastating like myasthenia gravis, polio, Guillain-Barre syndrome, muscular dystrophy, Amyotrophic Lateral Sclerosis (ALS) and others. These patients may need a ventilator when the condition is advanced. If disease can be treated or resolved, the ventilator can come off or perhaps, unfortunately, the ventilator may be used for the rest of the patient's life.

Ventilatory Failure Problem #5 - Pulmonary Blood Blocked from Reaching Ventilated Lung Tissue

This is hard to visualize: see the diagram at the end of Chapter 2. It is not that uncommon, but difficult to diagnose. The common onset is caused by a blood clot breaking loose from the legs and coming up through the heart and getting stuck blocking the blood vessels on the way to the lungs. A huge blood clot might block one or both lungs. Hemorrhagic pulmonary embolism, or a bunch of small clots (microembolism) may block many smaller branches of the blood vessels to the lungs. Pulmonary embolism can also be caused by air in the bloodstream (air embolism) or blobs of fat from long bone fractures (fatty emboli). These emboli block the blood from the air sacs, so no matter how much the patient ventilates the fresh air does not cross over to the blood. This is called wasted ventilation or deadspace ventilation. Regardless of the type of embolism the severity is usually dependent on the size of the blockage and if it can be reversed. A ventilator may be needed for the patient during diagnosis and treatment.

It is thought that some viruses, ex. Sars-cov-2, may cause swelling and inflammation of the smallest blood vessels in the lungs, the pulmonary capillaries. This swelling and inflammation may be a form of ARDS and be a very serious impediment to proper ventilation and oxygenation.

Oxygenation Failure

The patient in oxygenation failure is unable to get oxygen from the atmosphere into their blood. The problem is not that there is not enough oxygen in the atmosphere nor that the patient is not ventilating the oxygen down inside the lung, assuming ventilation is accomplished properly as described above. The oxygen problem is that venous blood needing oxygen coming back from the body comes to alveoli (air sacs) that are collapsed, partially ventilated, filled with liquid, or otherwise not fully functional with respect to having oxygen available for the blood. So, the blood passes through the lungs without getting fully oxygenated.

Oxygenation is assessed by measuring P_aO_2 by arterial blood gas analysis. Using a pulse oximeter measuring S_pO_2 is the easiest and next best.

Simplistically, if the results of the arterial blood gas sample taken to assess the initial settings has a P_aO_2 below normal limits (80 – 100 Torr.), we will change the F_IO_2 in mild cases requiring < 40 to 60% oxygen. Increasing F_IO_2 does not solve the underlying problem; just provides a high enough oxygen concentration that the blood will be adequately oxygenated in spite of the problem. If F_IO_2 > 40 – 60% is needed, usually the physician will apply more PEEP in 5 cmH_2O increments until an adequate P_aO_2 is reached. If the PEEP reaches 15 – 20 cmH$_2$O without achieving an adequate P$_a$O$_2$, usually the physician will increase the F$_I$O$_2$ into the toxic range up to 100% oxygen. So, the idea here is to use a minimal amount of oxygen if possible; if that doesn't work add PEEP; if the PEEP gets too high, then toxic levels have to be used to keep the patient alive. If all of this does not provide adequate P$_a$O$_2$ the patient is in a very difficult situation and any number of less usual strategies may be pursued.

The rationale for this process of normalizing P$_a$O$_2$ is relatively simple. Most physicians think that low levels of oxygen (F$_I$O$_2$ < 40 -60%) are safer than increasing PEEP above 5 - 10 cmH$_2$O. Likewise, most physicians think that 10 – 20 cmH$_2$O of PEEP is safer than F$_I$O$_2$ > 40 -60%. Finally, most physicians believe that increasing F$_I$O$_2$ > 40 -60% is a lesser evil than PEEP > 20 cmH$_2$O.

Complicating this scheme of managing oxygenation is that most physicians will tolerate wider limits for P$_a$O$_2$ for ventilator patients between 60 –120 mmHg. Also, some patients with COPD need to keep P$_a$O$_2$ in the range of 50 – 55 mmHg, because their chronic ventilatory failure has disrupted normal control of breathing in their brain. They need a lower blood oxygen to stimulate their breathing.

Ventilator Patient Management Problems

In General:

A very wise, old neonatologist, Robert A. DeLemos, MD once said:

"Ventilation can be understood by realizing that $\Delta P \sim P_aCO_2$", where Δ = change and P = pressure. This means that changes in the pressure in the airway causes air movement/breaths and that changes in P_aCO_2 are inversely proportional to the airway pressure changes or the number and size of the resulting breaths.

"Oxygenation can be understood by realizing that $MAP \sim P_aO_2$.", where MAP = mean airway pressure or arithmetic average airway pressure (meaning that as the average pressure in the airway increases, so will the P_aO_2 and vice versa, or P_aO_2 is directly proportional to MAP changes). If the ventilator gives deeper breaths, more breaths or more PEEP oxygenation will improve.

Let's explore this briefly.

$\Delta P \sim P_aCO_2$ - ΔP is the difference between baseline and peak airway pressure. ΔP is increased every time the peak airway pressure goes up or baseline pressure goes down. In almost every circumstance this will result in movement of air in or out of the lung. Respiratory rate is the number of breaths (ΔPs) per minute. Tidal volume is related to the magnitude of ΔP. The larger the ΔP the fewer are necessary to generate adequate minute volume and vice-versa. For example, in the two pressure vs. time waveforms from a ventilator display screen, the one on the top with 4 x 15 cmH_2O breaths should result in time about the same P_aCO_2 as the waveform on the bottom with 2 x 30 cmH$_2$0. This is a general rule, so we don't need to do the math, but they both equal about 60 cmH$_2$0 ~ ΔP.

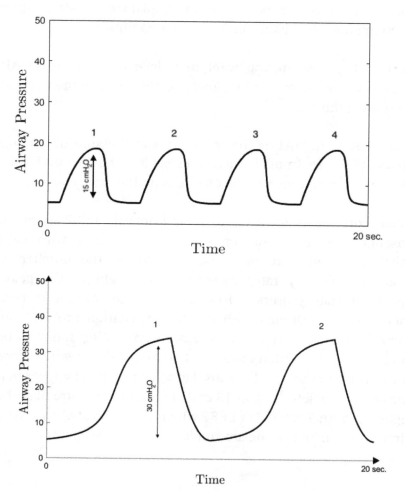

To some healthcare providers this concept is not obvious and changes to ventilator settings may be made that are not straightforward changes in respiratory rate or tidal volume that significantly effect ΔP ~ P$_a$CO$_2$.

There are few, if any, exceptions to this basic concept. It can be applied to VCV, PCV, APRV, Bi-level, HFJV, HFO. Sometimes it will appear that this is not true; however, in most every case that appearance can be reasonably explained by some other phenomenon or a change in the patient condition.

<u>Bottom Line</u>: When you want to reduce P_aCO_2 increase ΔP. This could be increasing PIP, lowering the baseline pressure, or increasing the rate.

MAP ~ P_aO_2 MAP is the Mean Airway Pressure or average airway pressure. In mathematical terms it is the area under the pressure/time curve. See the diagrams on the next page.

What contributes to MAP? MAP is primarily PEEP or raised baseline pressure; however, the pressure peaks with each inhalation contribute more significantly as the number of peaks (respiratory rate) increases, the height of the peaks (peak inspiratory pressure) increases, and as inspiratory time increases. For patients with severe oxygenation problems all these factors can increase or decrease oxygenation and must be considered and titrated carefully. Looking at the pressure/time waveforms on the ventilator display screen, it might appear that the one on the left PEEP of 15 cmH_2O is more pressure than the right one with 5 cmH_2O of PEEP when in fact the MAPs are very similar, if you look at the area under the pressure curves.

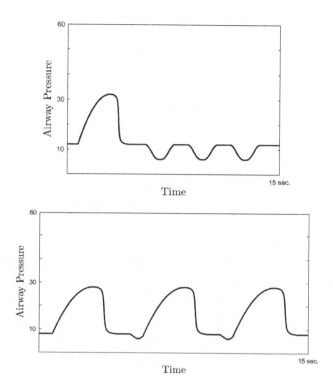

<u>Bottom Line</u>: When you want to increase P_aO_2 increase MAP. This could be increasing the PEEP/CPAP, increasing PIP, increasing inspiratory time and/or increasing respiratory rate. This is assuming that F_IO_2 is constant at a safe level or constant up to a maximum of 100%.

If the reader makes sense of this, you can understand anything in this book. No problem. If you can't make sense of this, I didn't explain it well enough.

Ventilator Patient Specific Problems and Possible Remedies

There are very many specific problems possible with the ventilator, the ventilator patient and the relationship between the two. This topic is long and tedious because of the complexity of the patient on one hand and the ventilator on the other.

A wise old respiratory therapist once said, "Being on a ventilator is about the most dangerous condition in the hospital."

It is more dangerous than surgery; because, in surgery, there is at least one surgeon and numerous nurses and other assistants present all the time. Ventilator patients are monitored electronically all the time, but the ICU nurse may have other patients, the physician may only visit once or twice a day and the respiratory therapist only comes by every 2 - 4 hours. Of course, if something bad happens the ventilator patient will have attention within a matter of seconds.

Patient's blood oxygen level is going down, and the oxygen percentage on the ventilator has to go up.

1. P_aO_2 is decreasing with increasing F_IO_2

What are we dealing with here?

The problem is almost always that the fresh air/oxygen from inhalation is not coming in contact with enough blood in the lungs to meet the body's needs. This happens when the alveoli get filled with fluids like pus or water leaking from the blood.

It could be collapse of the alveoli and small airways from inflammation or other similar pathology that keeps the air high in oxygen from coming in contact with the blood that is there to pick up the oxygen.

This is called "shunt". The blood is shunted from the right side of the heart (systemic venous blood needing oxygen) out through the lungs and back to the left side of the heart (systemic arterial blood) going out to the body without picking up enough oxygen. This is called "right-to- left intrapulmonary shunt."It is called intrapulmonary shunt because the "by-pass" occurs in the lungs or pulmonary area. When we measure this arterial blood for oxygen, it is low.

The illustration below shows R-L intrapulmonary shunt with blood coming to the lung unoxygenated (blue). The right side is working well with good ventilation and good blood flow. The left poorly ventilated alveolus is R-L intrapulmonary shunt. The shunted blood mixes in with the oxygenated blood and results in a decreased P_aO_2.

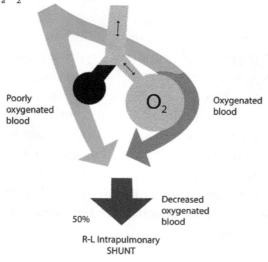

If we turn up the oxygen percentage in the inspired air in a right-to-left intrapulmonary shunt condition, it makes little or no difference; because the air going down into the lungs isn't getting to meet with the blood. So, it doesn't matter too much, whether it is just room air, 21% oxygen, or 60% oxygen. Either way it's simply not interfacing with the blood. In this case increasing the percentage of oxygen does not improve the arterial P_aO_2.

We say this P_aO_2 is refractory to changes in F_IO_2. We need to assess the situation and increase the patient's arterial blood oxygen in some other way.

The measurement of R-L intrapulmonary shunt is Q_S/Q_T, where Q is cardiac output, S is the shunted blood and T is total blood. Translated, we are measuring the percentage of blood going to the lung that is not meeting aerated lung tissue. In other words, we are measuring the efficiency of the lungs to deliver oxygen to the blood. The equation for Q_S/Q_T is:

$$C_cO_2 - CaO_2 / C_cO_2 - C_vO_2$$

Where "C" is oxygen content in milliliters per 100milliliters of blood, "c" is pulmonary capillary oxygen content (ml/dl), "a" is arterial oxygen content, and "v" is mixed venous oxygen content. Mixed venous blood is the blood going from the right heart to the lungs. It is a mixture of all the venous blood coming back from various parts of the body. Mixed venous blood is difficult to sample and requires the use of a pulmonary artery catheter (Swan-Ganz catheter) that has been placed through a major vein like the jugular, brachial, or femoral vein and "floated" back to the right heart, through the right heart and settled in the pulmonary artery.

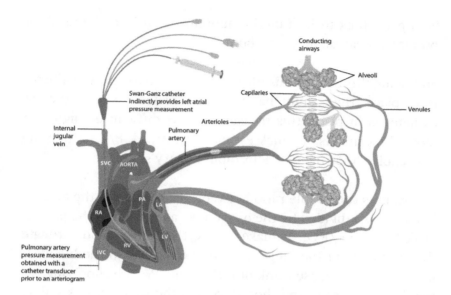

We need P_aO_2, S_aO_2, Hb, P_aCO_2, S_vO_2, P_vO_2, P_B to do this calculation. To have all these numbers simultaneous blood gas samples must be drawn from an artery as well as from a pulmonary artery catheter. Or we can get an arterial blood gas and a special oximetric pulmonary artery catheter will provide S_vO_2, but no P_vO_2. So, we just use $P_vO_2 = 40$ Torr. as a constant. Whether the P_vO_2 is 20 or 60 Torr is insignificant in the calculation of Q_S/Q_T. This calculation accurately measures the efficiency of the lungs to deliver oxygen to the blood.

If the reader thinks this is difficult to understand, it is. It is so difficult to understand that many practitioners don't completely understand it, and this is one reason that survival rate for ARDS on mechanical ventilation may be as low as it is. Scientific studies have been published that show the outcome of ARDS in equally sick patients is worse if they have a pulmonary artery catheter in place. Certainly, if the pulmonary artery catheter is not used optimally, its side-effects outweigh its value in understanding and treating ARDS. In some cases, the pulmonary artery catheter is in place for cardiac function monitoring and can be used for pulmonary calculations as a bonus.

Following through on this idea, if no pulmonary artery catheter is in place, then shunt has to be estimated. Even if the PA catheter is in place, this measurement is difficult enough that most clinicians use a quick estimation instead. P/F ratio is the best choice to estimate R-L intrapulmonary shunt.

P/F ratio is the simple ratio between the oxygen in the arterial blood (P_aO_2) divided by the oxygen we are giving to the patient (F_IO_2), so P_aO_2/F_IO_2. It makes sense that this should estimate the efficiency of the lungs in getting oxygen into the blood. If it doesn't make sense think of it this way. We are supplying "F" number of shoes to the shoe store and the shoe store is selling "P" number of shoes. This gives us an estimation of the efficiency of shoe sales in that shoe store by comparing sales to what they have available. Like the shoe store analogy this leaves out quite a few assumptions.

What is normal P_aO_2/F_IO_2? Normal P_aO_2 = 100 mmHg. Room air is 21% oxygen, so normal F_IO_2 = about 0.21 then 100/.21 = 476: therefore, normal P/F ratio = about 500. If the lungs worked perfectly, we could calculate by another method that ideal P/F ratio; would be about 600. However, our lungs are not ideal and have about 5 - 10% R-L intrapulmonary shunt normally.

The rule of the thumb for using P/F ratio is for every 100 change in P/F ratio is about 5% change in R-L intrapulmonary shunt. If P/F ratio is going down, the percent shunt is going up. It is an inverse relationship. If P/F ratio is decreasing, then shunt is increasing, and the patient is getting worse and therefore needing more oxygen. If the P/F ratio is increasing, then shunt is decreasing, and the patient is getting better; we are doing something right.

Just remember P/F ratio of 300 = 15% shunt,
  • for every 100 change in P/F ratio estimated shunt varies inversely by 5%
  • for every 20 change in P/F ratio estimated shunt varies inversely by 1%

  So...   P/F ratio of 200 = 20% shunt, 100 = 25% shunt
         P/F ratio of 400 = 10% shunt, 500 = 5% shunt

When the patient's P_aO_2 < 100 mmHg the estimation is less correct due to not taking hemoglobin into account. Q_s/Q_T does take hemoglobin into account. A good thing is that P/F ratio tends to underestimate shunt, so the medical team is not likely to respond with changes to overestimation. A P/F ratio <300 is one of the definitions of ARDS.

Let's look at a clinical example of a patient named Adam where the P_aO_2 = 88 mmHg. on 30% oxygen, F_IO_2 = 0.30, then P/F ratio is 88/0.30 = 293 or about 300. If P/F ratio is 300, so we have about 15% R-L intrapulmonary shunt. Although, a P_aO_2 = 88 mmHg is low normal on room air; it is not normal at all in this case because Adam is on more oxygen than usual (30% instead of 21%), and his lungs are sending 15% of the blood out to the body without coming in contact with oxygenated lung sacs.

In the paragraph above our patient meets the P/F ratio inclusion criteria for ARDS according to the ARDSNet Protocol. (see Chap 7) Now let's say Adam's condition gets worse where the P_aO_2 = 55 mmHg. on 40% oxygen, F_IO_2 = 0.40, then P/F ratio is 55/0.40 = 137. This would be a R-L intrapulmonary of about 25%, maybe

23%. The ventilator care team would need to focus on the cause of the shunt and treat it if possible and also have to increase oxygenation by adding more oxygen or PEEP.

Thorough assessment of oxygenation must go beyond the ventilator to include cardiac output, the amount of hemoglobin to carry the oxygen, and the body's demand for oxygen. To do this we must measure the amount of blood being pumped by the heart; as well as look at the mixed venous blood from all over the body coming back to the lungs. If the cardiac output is low, or the mixed venous blood has very low oxygen or is acidotic, those are signs of oxygenation problems caused by poor circulation.

Some normal values to reference

$Q = 5$ L/min. $S_aO_2 = 97\%$ $S_vO_2 = 75\%$
$P_vO_2 = 40$ Torr. $C_aO_2 = 20$ vol.% C_vO_2 = 15 vol.%
$avDO_2 = 5$ vols% $pH_v = 7.\,30 - 7.35$

2. P_aCO_2 is rising above 35 - 45 mmHg

If we want the P_aCO_2 to come down, we must supply more minute volume by increasing respiratory rate or tidal volume (increase ΔP).

Higher than normal P_aCO_2 is called hypercarbia or hypercapnia. The first choice to reverse hypercapnia is to increase the number of breaths by increasing the ventilator respiratory rate. If for some reason we think the tidal volume needs increasing, we might increase the ventilator volume which will increase the peak pressure. In a situation where the P_aCO_2 is rising or stays too high and the tidal volume, respiratory rate or the pressures cannot be increased, the physician may decide that "permissive hypercapnia" is the best strategy. Permissive hypercapnia strategy is essentially, "we can't fix it, so we are going to accept it and deal with the consequences like acidemia.

3. High peak inspiratory pressure

First, we look for the most obvious reason, that the patient is coughing. If so, we may need to help the patient deal with pulmonary secretions by suctioning them out of the airway. We need to listen to the chest for bronchospasm and use bronchodilator medication if necessary. We may need to check for irritation of airways as the ET tube is very uncomfortable. If the patient is awake, we may want to ask "Yes/No" questions to inquire about the problem. Sometimes we may need to use medications to reduce cough and irritation.

Second, is the patient out of synchrony with the ventilator? If so, we adjust the ventilator or help the patient relax. We look at the patient and look at the ventilator very closely. Is the patient trying to breathe out when the ventilator is giving a breath in? If so, we may change mode to include spontaneous breathing. Is the patient trying to breathe in and the ventilator is not responding? If so, we may increase the trigger sensitivity or change to a mode with spontaneous breathing.

Third, with a patient in a spontaneous breathing mode, is the ventilator meeting the patient's inspiratory demand? If it is not meeting the patient's needs, we may increase the rise time which accelerates the ventilator inspiratory flowrate to better satisfy the patient's demand. Is the patient trying to get a breath and the ventilator is still in expiratory time doing nothing? If so, we increase the expiratory trigger sensitivity (ETS), so the ventilator will be ready sooner for the patient's next breath.

Fourth, are any of the inspiratory tubes kinked, blocked or perhaps the patient is biting on the oral endotracheal tube? If so, we straighten out the tubing and/or place a bite block between the teeth to protect the endotracheal tube.

Fifth, is the patient's compliance going down (lungs and/or chest wall getting stiffer)? If so we need to find the cause of decreased compliance and reverse it.

Sixth, is the patient's airway resistance going up (airway obstruction or constriction)? If so, we need to determine the cause of increased airway resistance and reverse it. This might be as simple as clearing the airway with a suction catheter or administering a bronchodilator medicine. Look to see if the in-line suction catheter is down too far. If the staff fail to pull it all the way out, it can obstruct the airway.

Seventh, is the inspiratory peak flow too high? If the whole tidal volume is being pushed in faster than necessary, it will generate more pressure than necessary. If so, reduce the inspiratory flow rate and this will allow the tidal volume to go in over a little more time and reduce the spike in peak pressure.

Eighth, is the ventilator giving rapid breaths that are out of control? If the ventilator is auto-cycling at a high speed, or "chattering", usually reducing the trigger sensitivity will solve the problem.

Ninth, is the patient stacking breaths without much exhalation in between? If the patient is on assist-control mode and is initiating breaths, it is possible the patient is inhaling at a higher flowrate than the ventilator set inspiratory flowrate. This may cause the ventilator to trigger a second breath within the inspiratory phase of the first breath; thus, the patient gets a double breath. This is usually solved by increasing the ventilator inspiratory flowrate to greater than what the patient is pulling, or place the patient on a spontaneous mode, or sedate and paralyze the patient. The first two solutions are usually preferable to the third.

4. High mean airway pressure

First the respiratory therapist will look at the patient; then look at the ventilator and check whether it is a trend.

To assess this alarm condition further the respiratory therapist looks at the ventilator graphic on the ventilator display panel checking the pressure/volume loop for overdistention of the lungs and any unnecessary pressure being applied to the lungs. Please see the illustration below. Please note this is a pressure/volume curve. The bottom of the loop is inspiration from a low pressure of 10 cmH_2O up to a peak pressure of 40 cmH_2O. The top line of the loop is exhalation from 40 coming back down to 10. Check the P/V loop for lung opening pressure and over pressure "beaking." In the graph below this patient is on 10 cmH_2O PEEP, but the lung is open up at 15 -17 cmH_2O; see the arrow. In addition, at about 32 cmH_2O there is a "penguin beak" where the pressure goes up to 40 cmH_2O, but very little more tidal volume is going in the lungs. We could make the patient safer from VILI and the ventilator more efficient by increasing the PEEP to 15 cmH_2O and reducing P High to 32 cmH_2O. This might allow less pressure changes in the lung for about the same amount of tidal volume.

Overdistention

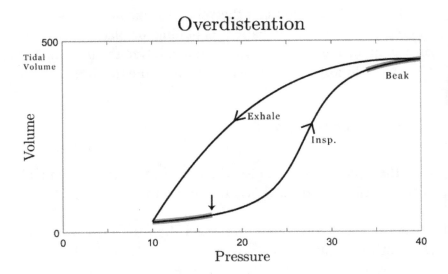

For further investigation the respiratory therapist will check the patient's compliance and if low, look for abdominal distention, often a swollen belly will push up against the diaphragm. Then look for fluid overload, often the patient is in kidney failure, or the IV fluids are going in too fast. Look for pulmonary edema, the patient may be in left heart failure or developing sepsis. It could be worsening ARDS or even seizures. Look for any new bandages or restraints that may be hindering chest movement.

In addition, the respiratory therapist will check the patient's airway resistance and if high, look for thick secretions partially blocking the artificial airway. Next, look for bronchospasm, often the person's airway muscles spasm and narrow the airway. Look further to see if the ET Tube is too small in diameter or there are other small lumen connectors in the patient breathing circuit.

It is also good to check the size of the tidal volume and look to see if the size of each breath can be reduced and lower the pressure.

The respiratory therapist needs to check the flow/time waveform, look to see if the shape of inspiratory phase of ventilation could be changed to patterns that generated less pressure. Different waveforms have different peak flows depending on the type of ventilator. If reasonable, change to a square or sinusoidal waveform that may deliver the breath with less pressure.

It is appropriate for the respiratory therapist to check the mode of ventilation; if the ventilator is controlling the patient or is assist-control mode with no spontaneous breathing, it may be appropriate to try a mode of ventilation that includes spontaneous breathing or try an automated mode where the ventilator itself can intelligently reduce the mean airway pressure.

5. Gasping for air

This miserable situation is not tolerable for the patient or the ventilator.

If the patient is gasping for air, increase the inspiratory flowrate, or decrease the trigger sensitivity for machine breaths to satisfy them. For spontaneous breathing decrease P_{ramp} or rise time or increase expiratory trigger sensitivity to help. A simple solution for patients on control or assist-control ventilation is to place them on a mode with spontaneous breathing or an automated ventilator protocol.

It is also possible that the patient is agitated, delirious or otherwise distraught and none of the above will work. If this is the case the patient will need to be reassured, receive pain medication or perhaps sedation.

6. Apnea

Apnea or absence of ventilation maybe the reason why the patient is on the ventilator and this is not unexpected.

However, if the patient is in a spontaneous mode where we expect them to be doing some breathing, and they are depending upon their own spontaneous respirations, then apnea is problematic.

First, we need to check the patient's chest and abdominal wall to see if they are trying to breathe and cannot pull in a breath because of some airway obstruction. This is usually not the case. If it is, the obstruction must be identified immediately and removed.

Second, we need to check if the P_aCO_2 level in the blood is too low. Low P_aCO_2 will not stimulate the brain to initiate spontaneous breathing, and the patient will become apneic. Here we want to reduce the amount of ventilation provided by the ventilator by turning down the respiratory rate.

Third, if the ventilator trigger sensitivity is too high, the patient cannot get a breath, so we will turn down trigger sensitivity and make it easier for the patient to trigger a breath.

Fourth, is a patient receiving too much sedation that is causing apnea, transient cessation of respiration?
. Too much sedation is not necessarily an error as sedatives affect some patients more than others, and can accumulate in patients over time; especially, when some older patients do not metabolize these drugs as fast as younger patients.

7. Tachypnea

Tachypnea means the patient is breathing too fast, usually more than 20 to 30 times per minute. People cannot reasonably breathe this fast and will tire out.

First, we check if the patient is anxious. If so, we will try to resolve their anxiety. This can be easy if the patient just wants something, and we can determine what it is and get it for them. It can be very difficult if the patient is delirious, combative or unreasonable, and sedation may have to be used.

Second, we check the patient's oxygen and carbon dioxide level and make sure they are normal. If the patient is short of oxygen or has a high carbon dioxide, this can stimulate them to breathe too fast. This can be resolved as described previously.

Third, check the patient's pH. If the pH is severely acidotic, the patient will be trying to breathe faster to blow off or reduce carbon dioxide that is being carried in the blood as carbonic acid. We will have to identify and resolve the acidosis in order to slow down the breathing.

Fourth, check the trigger sensitivity. If it is too sensitive, it can give the patient breaths very rapidly.

Fifth, if the patient is developing interstitial pulmonary capillary congestion, i.e., fluid or inflammation in the pulmonary capillary membrane, they may breathe shallow and rapidly. This is called the juxtapulmonary capillary receptor or J receptor reflex. It stimulates tachypnea. This is very hard to detect and if detected it is not certain to be the cause of tachypnea.

Tachypnea is one of the hardest problems for the ICU team to reverse if the patient just keeps breathing too fast. Cutting off the patient's air or stuffing a sock in their airway is just unacceptable. If the tachypnea cannot be slowed down, and it is detrimental to the patient, they may have to be sedated or placed in a "medical coma" with drugs.

8. Weak Inspiratory Effort

If the patient is in a mode with spontaneous breathing, their inspiratory efforts may need to be supported with a pressure boost from the machine. We will look at the patient; and then look at the ventilator

Is the patient sedated or paralyzed? If so, at least one reason is obvious.

We will check the P_aCO_2, and the patient's pH. If the P_aCO_2 is low, and the patient's pH is high they will both have the same diminishing effect on central control of breathing. This is especially true if the P_aO_2 is normal or high, so that the primary chemical stimulus to breathe is decreased and not backed up by hypoxic drive.

Of course, we will check trigger sensitivity to be sure it is not set too high.

At this point it might be ideal to place the patient on an automated mode that is monitoring the patient breath-to-breath for tidal volume, P_aCO_2, or neural signals from the diaphragm. This may allow the patient every opportunity to breathe spontaneously while protecting against hypoventilation.

9. Low exhaled tidal volume

Regardless of the mode of ventilation we will look at the patient, and the ventilator. Initially check the ventilator inspiratory tidal volume settings or measured values. The exhaled volumes should be about the same as the inspiratory volumes. If not, check for leaks in the patient tubing circuit, endotracheal tube cuff leaks, and other leaks including the chest tube if there is one in place. These mechanical leaks can be easily tightened and eliminated. If the leak is out of the chest tube, it means there is a hole in the lung through to the pleural space (bronchopleural fistula) and tidal volume is leaking out a hole in the lung to the chest tube evacuation system. If this is a large leak, it is serious and should be measured and monitored closely. Options for closing bronchopleural fistula are very difficult and hopefully it will heal shut on its own.

Measure tidal volume with another spirometer to check accurate measurements.

10. Auto-PEEP

What is Auto-PEEP, Inadvertent PEEP, Intrinsic PEEP?

It is air trapping in the patient's lungs when the next inspiration begins before the last breath was completely exhaled. The trapped air exerts a pressure deep in the lung; this is auto-PEEP.

Auto-PEEP is hidden PEEP. It does not appear on the pressure gauge, pressure monitor, or digital readout for PEEP; because those numbers come from the patient's upper airway at best or from the ventilator. Auto-PEEP is happening down inside the lung. So, to measure it we have to have some method to equilibrate lung pressure with our manometer or have a pleural catheter (an invasive catheter placed between the lungs' covering (visceral pleura) and the chest wall covering (parietal pleura).

Methods of <u>detecting</u> Auto-PEEP:

Look at the Flow/Time curve on the front display of the ventilator. Do not look at the manometer (pressure gauge) reading or the Pressure/Time curve. Do not look at the Volume/Time curve.

When looking at the Flow/Time curve below, check that the ascending end portion of the expiration curve (the dotted line below the zero baseline) meets the baseline, zero flow, prior to the inspiratory flow, which is the red line that starts above the baseline. If it does not, like the solid black expiratory curves, there is likely auto-PEEP. Unfortunately, we don't know how much.

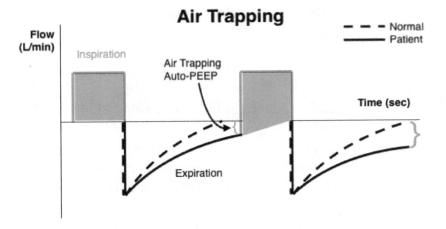

Another very esoteric method to detect Auto-PEEP is to check the expiratory time (T_E) and be sure it is at least 3 times the expiratory time constant (RC_{exp}). Most ventilators are not capable of measuring and reporting this value, but some ventilators do measure it. Many practitioners don't know how to use these numbers. However, this can be measured and calculated with standard hospital equipment.

What is a time constant? It is a noun. A time that represents the speed with which a particular system can respond to change, typically equal to the time taken for a specified parameter to vary by a factor of approximately 0.6321. It involves a differential equation concept that we don't need to discuss here, because RC_{exp} actually makes common sense when we use it as an example.

What is expiratory time constant (RC_{exp})? In words, it is a measure of how long it will take to empty the lungs by passive exhalation which is not linear. This will vary depending on how open or closed are the airways and how stiff or elastic is the chest wall.

Expiratory Time Constant (RC_{exp}) = Expiratory Resistance (R_{exp}) x Lung Thoracic Compliance (C_{LT})

Units for R_{exp} are = $cmH_2O/L/sec$
Normal values for R_{exp} are = 1 - 2 $cmH_2O/L/sec$

This means it takes a slight pressure difference, 1 - 2 cmH_2O for a normal person to breath out. This is just to overcome the resistance of the airways.

Units for C_{LT} are = L/cmH_2O
Normal values for C_{LT} are = 0.2 L/cmH_2O

This means it makes a slight pressure difference 0.1 - 0.5 cmH_2O when the lung and chest wall tissues recoil when breathing out.

When we multiply R_{exp} x C_{LT}, the L/cmH_2O cancel each other out, leaving seconds or time, as in time constant.

$RC_{exp} = (\text{cmH}_2\text{O/L/sec}) (\text{L/cmH}_2\text{O})$

Using normal values for resistance and compliance we can calculate expiratory time constant as below:

$RC_{exp} = (cmH_2O/L/sec) (L/cmH_2O)$
$RC_{exp} = (1\ cmH_2O/L/sec) (0.2\ L/cmH_2O)$

$RC_{exp} = \text{seconds}$
$RC_{exp} = 0.2\ \text{seconds}$

Ventilator patients are different from normal patients because they have respiratory illness, so probably their resistance and/ or compliance are not normal.

Using typical ventilator patient values for R_{exp} and C_{LT}, we might have:

$RC_{exp} = (22\ cmH_2O/L/sec) (0.04L/cmH_2O)$ or $RC_{exp} = 0.88$ seconds

Next we need to understand how to use time constants to detect Auto-PEEP.

Mathematically for each RC_{exp} there is a fixed percentage of V_T exhaled during the breath.

1 time constant = 63%
2 time constants = 87%
3 time constants = 95%
4 time constants = 98%

95% is enough for clinical purposes. Therefore, three time constants should be enough time for the patient to get almost all of their breath out each exhalation without air trapping and generating auto-PEEP. If the expiratory time is less than 3 time constants, we can expect to find air trapping in the lungs and pressure (auto-PEEP) building up out in the periphery of the lungs.

Looking at the normal example above 3 time constants = 0.3 secs. So, a normal person has plenty of time to exhale a normal breath.

Looking at the ventilator patient above 3 time constants = 2.64 secs. So, this ventilator needs close to 3 seconds to breath out. If the ventilator is set to give the next breath before 2.64 secs. auto-PEEP will be generated.

The time constant does not measure auto-PEEP but lets us know that we should expect to find it if we try to measure it or want to reduce it.

Methods of Measuring Auto-PEEP:

Hopefully, the $30,000 microprocessor ventilator measures it for you, and is reasonably accurate.

If not, it is possible to approximate auto-PEEP by occluding the exhalation valve at end-exhalation; thereby allowing the pressure deep in the lung to equilibrate with the airway. This is particularly difficult, if not impossible, in a spontaneously breathing patient. This difficulty is also why under certain conditions microprocessor ventilators cannot report the auto-PEEP value. It is better that the ventilator not report a grossly erroneous value if it can't measure it accurately.

It is usually desirable to reduce or eliminate auto-PEEP when present, whether we have been able to measure it or not.

Methods of reducing Auto-PEEP

1. Increase expiratory time; this allows the patient to breathe out longer and not trap air.
2. Decrease inspiratory time; this may by default increase expiratory time, see #1 above.
3. Reduce respiratory rate; if I/E ratio is the same, this increases expiratory time, see #1 above.
4. Reduce expiratory resistance (R_{exp}) by suctioning the patient, this opens the airway and allows higher expiratory flowrate, so the exhaled air gets out faster
5. Reduce R_{exp} by administering bronchodilators/anti-inflammatories; same result as #4
6. Reduce R_{exp} by changing imposed WOB, ex. tiny adapters, ET Tube; same result as #4

One could reduce auto-PEEP by decreasing compliance, but that is usually not the reason for auto-PEEP and is seldom a good idea.

Preventing auto-PEEP is a constant monitoring activity making sure the patient has enough exhalation time and keeping airway resistance minimal.

Lung Recruitment Procedure

When a patient is extremely sick with a very low P/F ratio indicating much of the lung tissue is collapsed or filled with fluid, it might be wise to try to "recruit" or open some of the closed alveoli. We usually choose to do this when the oxygen is 60% or above and the PEEP = 15 - 20 cmH$_2$0 at which is a point we want to avoid Ventilator Induced Lung Injury (VILI). It has been shown that patients with low P/F ratio, increased V$_D$/V$_T$, and decreased compliance are the better candidates for recruitment maneuvers.

It might not be wise to do lung recruitment on some patients because they cannot tolerate the high pressures and the inspiratory hold during the ventilator inspiration. Some clinicians think that lung recruitment is a hazardous waste of time.

Lung recruitment is most often discussed and applied to patients with ARDS.

Lung recruitment is accomplished by applying much higher air pressure to the lungs for a short time and then increasing the PEEP to keep any recruited lung units recruited with the high pressure open. These maneuvers must be done with caution in patients with tenuous blood pressure, or chest tubes, and cannot be done in uncooperative spontaneously breathing patients.

Sophisticated microprocessor-controlled ventilators have built-in lung recruitment tools. A common one allows the operator to:

1. Set a beginning PEEP to start the maneuver, usually the current PEEP level.
2. Set a top pressure (P$_{top}$); perhaps 40 cmH$_2$O is used, up to 60 cmH$_2$O for patients with very stiff lungs.
3. Set end PEEP: PEEP at the end of recruitment maneuver. Usually 2 - 5 cmH$_2$O higher than beginning PEEP to keep any recruited lung open.
4. Set ramp speed, perhaps, 2 to 5 cmH$_2$O/sec. This is how fast the ventilator will increase the pressure from

beginning PEEP to P_{top}. If the patient is expected to tolerate the maneuver well a slower ramp speed may be used.

5. Set Pause time (T_{pause}). This is the length of time the ventilator will hold the patient at P_{top}. The optimal duration for top pressure is 10 secs. A shorter T_{pause} may be chosen for a less stable patient.

In the first screen shot below you can see the control settings to prepare for lung recruitment. In the second screen shot you can see the rather complicated results.

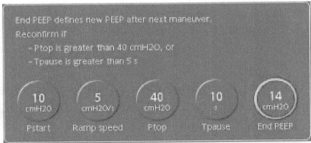

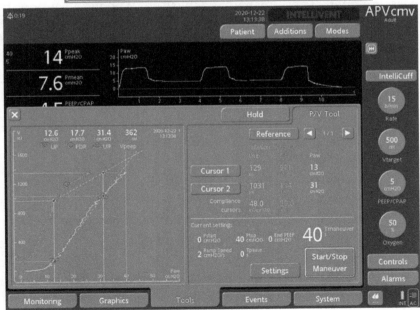

The process of lung recruitment gives the ICU physician and team additional information about the nature of the patient's ARDS.

There are other similar techniques for the lung recruitment involving stepwise increases and decreases in pressure to a high level temporarily. The basic concept is the same.

Lung recruitment may be attempted by prone positioning (face down) the patient. This is not as simple as it sounds since the patient is very sick and has many tubes and lines connected that we don't want pulled out. This requires several staff members to be present to safely turn the patient over. There are special, very expensive beds the hospital can purchase or rent to make this much easier. By turning the chest upside down the effects of gravity on lung tissue can "pull open" areas of the lungs that were in a dependent position while lying supine, face up.

Lung recruitment may be accomplished by using airway pressure relief ventilation (APRV) mode where the P_{high} is raised temporarily to a much higher level. The advantage of this is the patient is allowed to breathe spontaneously at P_{high}, and at P_{low} if reasonably possible. With APRV lung recruitment the PEEP may be increased after the recruitment maneuver to maintain any newly opened lung units.

CHAPTER 7

Ventilator Protocols and Standards of Care

This chapter is a collection of dissimilar topics that have best medical practices in common. Some like the ARDSNet protocol and spontaneous breathing trials are National and international methods that are backed by a significant amount of medical science research studies. There are National and International guidelines for only select aspects of care of patients on mechanical ventilators. These protocols have been in use for several years. Other methods, maneuvers, bundles, etc. described here are evidence-based practices with less high-level evidence but seem to be the best way to operate ventilators at this time.

   a. The ARDSNet protocol which provides guidance to the diagnosis and management of ventilator patients with ARDS
   b. Spontaneous Breathing Trial which is currently the best method of ventilator weaning
   c. Ventilator Bundle which was generated by the Institute for Healthcare Improvement (IHI) for the reduction of ventilator-associated pneumonia, infection, or "events".

d. Ventilator Associated Event/Ventilator Associated Pneumonia Prevention from the Centers for Disease Control and Prevention (CDC)

e. RCP driven protocols, American Association for Respiratory Care (AARC)

f. Quality Improvement

ARDSNet Protocol

The ARDSNet protocol is named after the largest U.S. government funded ventilator research project in history. They looked at the use of smaller tidal volumes, 6 ml/Kg. body weight. vs. larger tidal volumes of 12 ml/Kg. body weight for patients with ARDS. This study concluded that the smaller tidal volume, 6 ml./Kg., group had a lower mortality among ARDS patients. Both groups were on volume-assist-control mode of ventilation and were not allowed to breathe spontaneously unless during weaning trials.

Unfortunately, these results have been generalized to all ventilator patients regardless of disease entity or modes of ventilation. In other words they studied ARDS patients; therefore, the results apply only to ARDS patients. They studied only patients on assist-control, mode ventilation; therefore, the results apply only to patients on assist-control mode. Good application of science suggests it is not appropriate to generalize these results to all modes of ventilation nor to diseases other than ARDS.

Regardless, of any shortcomings of the research the follow-up was robust, and the ARDSNet Protocol was developed and refined and expanded over the ensuing years. The broad adoption of the ARDSNet protocol may have led to excessive use of the AC mode of ventilation and low tidal volumes in cases where deeper understanding of the patient's pathophysiology may have suggested other alternatives. As a result, this study may have contributed to the lack of progress in getting better survival for patients with ARDS for the last 20 years.

Please refer to the attached protocol card below to better understand the following explanations.

"Inclusion Criteria" is a definition of ARDS which delineates which ventilator patients should be treated with this protocol. The $PaO_2/FIO_2 \geq 300$ is a great criterion that encourages intervention in ARDS patients with an estimated R - L intrapulmonary shunt of about 15% or greater. The x-ray criteria describe ARDS well. The caveat, "No clinical evidence of left atrial hypertension" is to exclude a heart problem that mimics the first criteria but is most likely treated with cardiac and circulatory system medications.

"Ventilator Setup and Adjustment" is clear and important for initiation of ventilation and the protocol. This should be understandable to those who have read previous chapters of this book.

These are followed by ventilator management goals for "Oxygenation", "Plateau Pressure", "pH", and "I:E Ratio".

"Oxygenation Goal" is an attempt to reduce VILI by keeping the PEEP as low as possible while reducing oxygen toxicity by keeping the percent oxygen as low as possible. This "higher/ lower" method is not required.

"Plateau Pressure Goal" is an attempt to monitor lung-thoracic compliance and prevent VILI from high airway pressures.

"pH Goal" suggests that it is tolerable to breathe the patients at high respiratory rates to bring the pH up from acidosis by hyperventilating the patient or bringing the $PaCO_2$ below normal.

Part II of the protocol is a very specific method to perform weaning via spontaneous breath trial (SBT). It begins with Section A, specific criteria that indicate the patient may be ready to come off the ventilator and breathe spontaneously. Section B defines the method of SBT including section #1, that allows for three different apparatus for spontaneous breathing. The first two "T-piece" and "Trach collar" are essentially the same wherein the patient is taken off the ventilator entirely with a wish of good luck and hope of success while being monitored closely. Since CPAP and pressure support are removed the patient may experience some lung collapse and increased work of breathing due to the artificial airways still being in place. Regardless, it is a good pulmonary stress test and if the patient tolerates this for > 30 mins., they are possibly ready to breathe on their own and have the artificial airways removed. The third method is to leave the patient on the ventilator with minimal CPAP and pressure support in a spontaneous breathing mode. This helps the patient to avoid possible problems of spontaneous breathing with a tracheal tube; however, it adds the potential problem of how the ventilator provides spontaneous ventilation. Ventilators are engineered differently and spontaneous breathing on one brand of ventilator may be more or less work of breathing than another. Any of the three methods provide the patient a chance to try breathing on their own and to see if they are successful.

NIH NHLBI ARDS Clinical Network
Mechanical Ventilation Protocol Summary

OXYGENATION GOAL: PaO$_2$ 55-80 mmHg or SpO$_2$ 88-95%
Use a minimum PEEP of 5 cm H$_2$O. Consider use of incremental FiO$_2$/PEEP combinations such as shown below (not required) to achieve goal.

Lower PEEP/higher FiO2

FiO$_2$	0.3	0.4	0.4	0.5	0.5	0.6	0.7	0.7
PEEP	5	5	8	8	10	10	10	12

FiO$_2$	0.7	0.8	0.9	0.9	0.9	1.0
PEEP	14	14	14	16	18	18-24

Higher PEEP/lower FiO2

FiO$_2$	0.3	0.3	0.3	0.3	0.3	0.4	0.4	0.5
PEEP	5	8	10	12	14	14	16	16

FiO$_2$	0.5	0.5-0.8	0.8	0.9	1.0	1.0
PEEP	18	20	22	22	22	24

INCLUSION CRITERIA: Acute onset of
1. PaO$_2$/FiO$_2$ ≤ 300 (corrected for altitude)
2. Bilateral (patchy, diffuse, or homogeneous) infiltrates consistent with pulmonary edema
3. No clinical evidence of left atrial hypertension

PART I: VENTILATOR SETUP AND ADJUSTMENT
1. Calculate predicted body weight (PBW)
   Males = 50 + 2.3 [height (inches) - 60]
   Females = 45.5 + 2.3 [height (inches) -60]
2. Select any ventilator mode
3. Set ventilator settings to achieve initial V$_T$ = 8 ml/kg PBW
4. Reduce V$_T$ by 1 ml/kg at intervals ≤ 2 hours until V$_T$ = 6ml/kg PBW.
5. Set initial rate to approximate baseline minute ventilation (not > 35 bpm).
6. Adjust V$_T$ and RR to achieve pH and plateau pressure goals below.

PLATEAU PRESSURE GOAL: ≤ 30 cm H$_2$O
Check Pplat (0.5 second inspiratory pause), at least q 4h and after each change in PEEP or V$_T$.
If Pplat > 30 cm H$_2$O: decrease V$_T$ by 1ml/kg steps (minimum = 4 ml/kg).
If Pplat < 25 cm H$_2$O and V$_T$< 6 ml/kg, increase V$_T$ by 1 ml/kg until Pplat > 25 cm H$_2$O or V$_T$ = 6 ml/kg.
If Pplat < 30 and breath stacking or dys-synchrony occurs: may increase V$_T$ in 1ml/kg increments to 7 or 8 ml/kg if Pplat remains ≤ 30 cm H$_2$O.

pH GOAL: 7.30-7.45
Acidosis Management: (pH < 7.30)
If pH 7.15-7.30: Increase RR until pH > 7.30 or PaCO$_2$ < 25 (Maximum set RR = 35).

If pH < 7.15: Increase RR to 35.
If pH remains < 7.15, V$_T$ may be increased in 1 ml/kg steps until pH > 7.15 (Pplat target of 30 may be exceeded).
May give NaHCO$_3$
Alkalosis Management: (pH > 7.45) Decrease vent rate if possible.

I: E RATIO GOAL: Recommend that duration of inspiration be ≤ duration of expiration.

PART II: WEANING
A. Conduct a SPONTANEOUS BREATHING TRIAL daily when:
1. FiO$_2$ ≤ 0.40 and PEEP ≤ 8 OR FiO$_2$ ≤ 0.50 and PEEP ≤ 5.
2. PEEP and FiO$_2$ ≤ values of previous day.
3. Patient has acceptable spontaneous breathing efforts. (May decrease vent rate by 50% for 5 minutes to detect effort.)
4. Systolic BP ≥ 90 mmHg without vasopressor support.
5. No neuromuscular blocking agents or blockade.

B. SPONTANEOUS BREATHING TRIAL (SBT):
If all above criteria are met and subject has been in the study for at least 12 hours, initiate a trial of UP TO 120 minutes of spontaneous breathing with FiO2 ≤ 0.5 and PEEP ≤ 5:
1. Place on T-piece, trach collar, or CPAP ≤ 5 cm H$_2$O with PS ≤ 5
2. Assess for tolerance as below for up to two hours
   a. SpO$_2$ ≥ 90: and/or PaO$_2$ ≥ 60 mmHg
   b. Spontaneous V$_T$ ≥ 4 ml/kg PBW
   c. RR ≤ 35/min
   d. pH ≥ 7.3
   e. No respiratory distress (distress= 2 or more)
      ➢ HR > 120% of baseline
      ➢ Marked accessory muscle use
      ➢ Abdominal paradox
      ➢ Diaphoresis
      ➢ Marked dyspnea
3. If tolerated for at least 30 minutes, consider extubation.
4. If not tolerated resume pre-weaning settings.

Definition of **UNASSISTED BREATHING**
(Different from the spontaneous breathing criteria as PS is not allowed)

1. Extubated with face mask, nasal prong oxygen, or room air, OR
2. T-tube breathing, OR
3. Tracheostomy mask breathing, OR
4. CPAP less than or equal to 5 cm H$_2$O without pressure support or IMV assistance.

ARDSNet protocol ends with a strange black box that defines "Unassisted Breathing" a term that is not used on the ARDSNet protocol card at all. It seems to harken back in time to a bias against the use of IMV (intermittent mandatory ventilation). IMV that is not synchronized with the patient is almost never used these days. SIMV (synchronized intermittent mandatory ventilation) however, is used and is an essential part of almost all of the newer modes of ventilation including all highly automated ventilator protocols.

Spontaneous Breathing Trial (SBT)

Spontaneous Breathing Trial with a sedation "vacation" should be performed on patients daily if they meet assessment criteria for ventilator discontinuation. The usual practice is to perform SBT every morning on all ventilator patients who will not be harmed by the procedure. It makes sense to reduce the patient's sedation, so they will be able to breathe on their own.

The following chart is the recent Best Practice of the American Association for Respiratory Care. It follows the best practices outlined in publications of the American Thoracic Society and the American College of Chest Physicians. This guideline includes discussion of extubation and follow-up for patients successfully discontinued from the ventilator. This best practice is not nearly as specific as the ARDSNet SBT guideline and does not recommend the use of T-Piece/Trach collar weaning; however, this AARC best-practice avoids clear definition of the specific method of the SBT experience.

Issue	Best-Practice Description	Importance
Daily assessment for liberation potential	An assessment should be conducted at least daily to determine whether the patient meets criteria to move forward in the liberation process. The criteria might include: evidence of reversal of the underlying cause of respiratory failure, adequate oxygenation on PEEP <8 and FiO2 <0.50, hetmodynamic stability, and ability to initiate an inspiratory effort.	More than 70% of patients are successfully liberated following their initial SBT, suggesting that identifying the earliest point in time to conduct the SBT is important
SBT	Once meeting the liberation criteria, a spontaneous breathing trial (SBT) should be conducted before determining whether extubation can occur. Generally, the SBT should last 30-120 minutes.	Multiple studies have shown that the SBT should be the test to determine whether a patient is ready to assume breathing without assistance.
Linking SAT and SBT	Nursing should follow a sedation protocol. Therapists should conduct the SBT while the patient is undergoing a sedation awakening trial (SAT).	Conducting the SBT while the patient is minimally sedated has been associated with improved outcomes, including reduced mortality.

SBT Failure	Generally, if the patient fails the SBT, he or she should be placed back on previous settings or a comfortable level of pressure support and reassessed the following day for liberation potential.	When patients have declared they are not ready to be liberated, pushing them further may impose excessive load on their respiratory system and can delay liberation or extend duration of invasive ventilation.

| Cuff leak test pre-extubation | Prior to extubation, in adults who have met extubation criteria AND are deemed high risk for post-extubation stridor (PES) (e.g., traumatic intubation, intubation >6 days, large endotracheal tube, female, reintubation after an unplanned extubation), a cuff leak test should be performed. If there is insufficient leak (failed test), it is recommended that systemic steroids be administered at least 4 hours before extubation. A repeat cuff leak test prior to extubation is not required. | Patients with PES have increased risk for reintubation, which itself is associated with increased morbidity and mortality. Identifying these patients is important so they can be treated prior to extubation. On the other hand, the cuff leak test is associated with a significant number of false negatives (i.e., fail test due to lack of leak, but do not have PES), which might unnecessarily delay extubation. The test should be reserved for patients at high risk for PES and not be conducted on all patients. |

| Prophy-lactic NIV post-extubation | For patients ventilated for >24 hours who pass an SBT AND are at high risk for extubation failure (e.g., patient with hypercarbia, COPD, CHF, or other co-morbidities), apply preventive NIV following extubation. It is recommended to apply NIV immediately after extubation to realize outcome benefits. | Patients who satisfactorily tolerate an SBT and require reintubation following extubation have increased risk for complications, including increased mortality. Use of preventive NIV in these high-risk patients, especially in COPD, is associated with a 14% relative increase in extubation success, and a relative reduction in ICU mortality of 63%. |

Please see Chapter 8 Ventilator Weaning for an in-depth discussion of weaning assessment and other weaning protocols.

Ventilator Bundle

The ventilator bundle is a collection of evidence-based ventilator patient care strategies to reduce the chance of the patient developing pneumonia or other untoward events as a result of being on a ventilator in ICU.

The current 2020 best standards are listed below:

1. Elevate the head of the bed (HOB) to between 30-45 degrees (use visual cues, designate one person to check for HOB every one to two hours). This helps prevent gastric juices and upper airway secretions from going down in the lungs.
2. Establish a process to perform routine oral care every two hours with antiseptic mouthwash and Chlorhexidine 0.12 percent every 12 hours. This cleans germs out of the mouth that could go down into the lungs.
3. Include peptic ulcer disease prophylaxis (PUD) on ICU admission orders and ventilator order sets as an automatic order that requires the physician to actively exclude it. Ventilator patients are prone to developing a stomach ulcer. This is meant to reduce the chance of that.
4. Include venous thromboembolism (VTE) prophylaxis on ICU admission orders and ventilator order sets as an automatic order that would require the physician to actively exclude it. VTE, blood clots, often occur in the leg veins when a patient is immobile. If these break loose, they will float back to the heart which could be problematic or pass on through the heart to certainly lodge in the increasingly small branching of the pulmonary arteries. Meaning they will lodge and plug up blood flow to the lungs. That creates pulmonary embolism and alveolar deadspace ventilation.

5. Invite families to participate in care by encouraging them to ask if prevention efforts have been completed, such as oral care and HOB elevation. Educate families on the risk of VAE, preventive measures put in place and what they can do to help (e.g., perform oral care or passive range of motion exercises if willing).

6. Perform and coordinate SAT (spontaneous awakening trial), sometimes called "sedation Vacation" and SBT (spontaneous breathing trial) to maximize weaning opportunities when patient sedation is minimal. Coordinate between nursing and respiratory therapy to manage SAT and SBT, perform daily assessment or readiness to wean and extubate.

7. Establish a process for timely physical and occupational therapy evaluation for patients on ventilator support to establish a plan for progressive mobility. With careful attention to detail some ventilators patients can exercise in bed, sit up on the bedside, or even go for a short walk.

8. Sedation should be goal oriented and should be administered, as ordered, by the physician according to a scale such as Richmond Agitation Sedation Scale (RASS). As can be easily imagined, over sedation and under sedation are both problematic.

VAE and VAP Prevention

VAE stands for "Ventilator Associated Event" which is a term invented by the CDC to try to make sense of a real, but poorly defined problem of VAP, "Ventilator Associated Pneumonia". The basic problem here is when patients are on ventilators their normal cough mechanism, upper airway filtering and air conditioning of inhaled air is compromised. In addition, they can be exposed to hospital bacteria and other germs that might not be found elsewhere. This problem gained attention in the early

2000s. The CDC started requiring hospitals to report a VAP rate which was the number of VAP cases per 1000 days of mechanical ventilation (VAP/1000 vent. days.). A day of mechanical ventilation is a day when there is a patient on a ventilator. This was a great idea, but problematic; because, as you can see in the algorithm below, the definition of a VAP case is very complex, and that is the numerator of the VAP rate. So, to further clarify this situation the CDC added the VAC, IVAC and PVAP terms in the flowchart below. See the definitions in the algorithm below. Whether or not this is clearer is clearly debatable.

In addition, the definition of a "ventilator day" is still not precisely defined, so the denominator is not a solid number. The standard method of counting ventilator days is highly variable depending on how it is done, or more specifically what time of day it is done. A good method for doing this will be discussed under Ventilator Quality of Care later in this chapter.

VAC/VAE/IVAC/VAP/PVAP prevention remains a laudable goal and in time the CDC will get the ambiguities out of the definitions of the numerator and denominator. The CDC focusing on the problem thus far has undoubtedly saved many lives.

Please see the "Ventilator-Associated Events (VAE) Surveillance Algorithm" on the next page.

Figure 1: Ventilator-Associated Events (VAE) Surveillance Algorithm

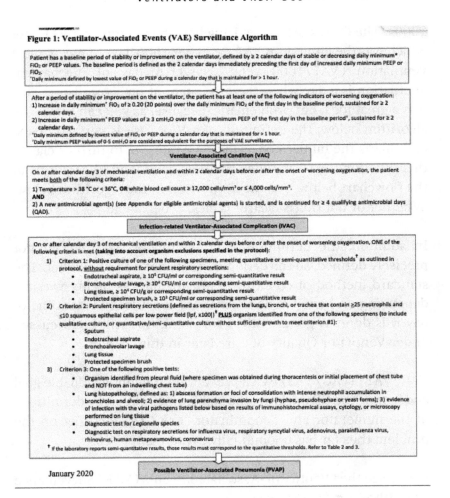

Patient has a baseline period of stability or improvement on the ventilator, defined by ≥ 2 calendar days of stable or decreasing daily minimum* FiO_2 or PEEP values. The baseline period is defined as the 2 calendar days immediately preceding the first day of increased daily minimum PEEP or FiO_2.
*Daily minimum defined by lowest value of FiO_2 or PEEP during a calendar day that is maintained for > 1 hour.

After a period of stability or improvement on the ventilator, the patient has at least one of the following indicators of worsening oxygenation:
1) Increase in daily minimum* FiO_2 of ≥ 0.20 (20 points) over the daily minimum FiO_2 of the first day in the baseline period, sustained for ≥ 2 calendar days.
2) Increase in daily minimum* PEEP values of ≥ 3 cmH_2O over the daily minimum PEEP of the first day in the baseline period†, sustained for ≥ 2 calendar days.
*Daily minimum defined by lowest value of FiO_2 or PEEP during a calendar day that is maintained for > 1 hour.
†Daily minimum PEEP values of 0-5 cmH_2O are considered equivalent for the purposes of VAE surveillance.

Ventilator-Associated Condition (VAC)

On or after calendar day 3 of mechanical ventilation and within 2 calendar days before or after the onset of worsening oxygenation, the patient meets **both** of the following criteria:

1) Temperature > 38 °C or < 36°C, **OR** white blood cell count ≥ 12,000 cells/mm^3 or ≤ 4,000 cells/mm^3.
AND
2) A new antimicrobial agent(s) (see Appendix for eligible antimicrobial agents) is started, and is continued for ≥ 4 qualifying antimicrobial days (QAD).

Infection-related Ventilator-Associated Complication (IVAC)

On or after calendar day 3 of mechanical ventilation and within 2 calendar days before or after the onset of worsening oxygenation, ONE of the following criteria is met **(taking into account organism exclusions specified in the protocol)**:

1) Criterion 1: Positive culture of one of the following specimens, meeting quantitative or semi-quantitative thresholds† as outlined in protocol, **without** requirement for purulent respiratory secretions:
   - Endotracheal aspirate, ≥ 10^5 CFU/ml or corresponding semi-quantitative result
   - Bronchoalveolar lavage, ≥ 10^4 CFU/ml or corresponding semi-quantitative result
   - Lung tissue, ≥ 10^4 CFU/g or corresponding semi-quantitative result
   - Protected specimen brush, ≥ 10^3 CFU/ml or corresponding semi-quantitative result
2) Criterion 2: Purulent respiratory secretions (defined as secretions from the lungs, bronchi, or trachea that contain ≥25 neutrophils and ≤10 squamous epithelial cells per low power field (lpf, x100))† **PLUS** organism identified from one of the following specimens (to include qualitative culture, or quantitative/semi-quantitative culture without sufficient growth to meet criterion #1):
   - Sputum
   - Endotracheal aspirate
   - Bronchoalveolar lavage
   - Lung tissue
   - Protected specimen brush
3) Criterion 3: One of the following positive tests:
   - Organism identified from pleural fluid (where specimen was obtained during thoracentesis or initial placement of chest tube and NOT from an indwelling chest tube)
   - Lung histopathology, defined as: 1) abscess formation or foci of consolidation with intense neutrophil accumulation in bronchioles and alveoli; 2) evidence of lung parenchyma invasion by fungi (hyphae, pseudohyphae or yeast forms); 3) evidence of infection with the viral pathogens listed below based on results of immunohistochemical assays, cytology, or microscopy performed on lung tissue
   - Diagnostic test for *Legionella* species
   - Diagnostic test on respiratory secretions for influenza virus, respiratory syncytial virus, adenovirus, parainfluenza virus, rhinovirus, human metapneumovirus, coronavirus

† If the laboratory reports semi-quantitative results, those results must correspond to the quantitative thresholds. Refer to Table 2 and 3.

January 2020

Possible Ventilator-Associated Pneumonia (PVAP)

Respiratory Care Practitioner (RCP) driven protocols

A respiratory care practitioner (RCP) is the professional name for a respiratory therapist. It was established when respiratory therapy became a licensed profession across the USA.

RCP driven protocols are a number of protocols that respiratory therapists, physicians, nurses and hospitals have negotiated to allow the respiratory therapist to use their knowledge and skills more independently. The value of this is better patient care and better communication among health care professionals.

The RCP driven protocol for mechanical ventilation is the RCP driven protocol of interest here.

Instead of ordering all the ventilator parameters the ER physician or intensivist may order: "Ventilator Protocol"

SAMPLE RCP VENTILATOR PROTOCOL:

1. Conduct patient assessment prior to use of a mechanical ventilator
   a. CPR Code status/Advanced Directives
   b. Alternatives to CMV, consider CPAP or BiPAP
   c. Airway patency
      i. endotracheal or tracheostomy tube placement verified
      ii. bilateral breath sounds
      iii. adequate gas exchange with hand ventilation
   d. Spontaneous respiratory drive (present or absent)
   e. Chest drainage system patency
   f. Arterial blood gas results or reliable S_pO_2 /$ETCO_2$ data, if possible
2. Set up and check the function of all equipment
   g. Ventilator circuit and/or in-line suction will be changed between patients and when soiled.
3. Initial ventilator settings/management:
   a. Mode: VCV (SIMV or AC) Adaptive Support Ventilation may be used

b. f: 6 – 20/min. allowing for adequate minute volume and patient's condition

c. V_T: 6 – 12 ml/Kg. ideal body weight

d. F_IO_2: 1.0 or adjusted appropriately according to oxygenation monitoring results

e. PEEP: 8.0 cmH$_2$O, where appropriate

f. PS: 5-15 cmH$_2$O as indicated

g. Other ventilator controls and alarm settings will be adjusted to optimize the patient/ventilator interface.

h. Documentation of initial patient assessment, ventilator settings and patient response will be entered on the ventilator flowsheet.

4. ABG may be drawn and analyzed approximately 10 minutes after initiation of mechanical ventilation ETCO$_2$ and S$_p$O$_2$ will be correlated with ABG values, if possible.

5. Management of patient/ventilator relationship. If the patient requires support outside these limits, consult with a physician.

a. Oxygenation

   i. Maintain S$_p$O$_2$ > 93% keeping FIO$_2$ < 0.6

   ii. Maintain PEEP $\leq$ 15 cm H$_2$O

   iii. Keep PEEP and FIO$_2$ as low as possible if SPO$_2$ > 93%. If P$_a$O$_2$ > 200 Torr. on F$_I$O$_2$ 1.0, change F$_I$O$_2$ to 0.6. Otherwise make F$_I$O$_2$ changes in increments of 0.1 (10%). Make PEEP changes in increments of 2 - 5 cmH$_2$O.

   iv. Monitor R-L intrapulmonary shunt, SvO$_2$, hemoglobin and cardiac output whenever practical

   v. Determine the cause of poor oxygenation and address other therapy to the cause/s.

b. Ventilation

   i. Maintain P$_a$CO$_2$ by changing respiratory frequency; make frequency changes in increments of 2 breaths/min.

    ii. Use correlated $ETCO_2$ to monitor frequency changes whenever possible

    iii. Maintain P_aCO_2 between 35 – 45 mmHg. keeping pH 7.30 – 7.45

    iv. Monitor resistance, lung-thorax compliance and deadspace to tidal volume ratio

    v. Determine the causes of increased resistance and decreased compliance and address other therapy to the cause/s.

  c. Reduction of work of breathing

    i. Adjust flow or pressure sensitivity for optimal initiation of inspiratory phase

    ii. Adjust flowrate, waveforms, and other adjuncts to optimize patient comfort

    iii. Reduce "mechanical" airway resistance

    iv. Evaluate "auto-PEEP"

    v. Add pressure support to overcome inspiratory resistance; make pressure support changes in increments of 5 cmH_2O

    vi. Increase expiratory time for patients with COPD and asthma

  d. Protection of the airways and lung parenchyma

    i. Maintain PIP < 60 cmH_2O

    ii. Maintain F_IO_2 < 0.6

    iii. Set appropriate alarms and limits in accordance with the patient's condition

  e. ABGs may be done as appropriate with each ventilator setting change or as warranted by the patient's clinical status.

6. Discontinuation of CMV

  a. Daily spontaneous breathing trial

    i. Nurse will withhold or reduce paralytic drugs or sedation as appropriate

   ii. Place the patient in spontaneous mode with PEEP $\leq$ 5 cmH$_2$O and PSV = 5 cmH$_2$O

   iii. Respiratory therapist to remain at the bedside monitoring the patient for the first 10 min.

   iv. Terminate the trial if, f > 35/min x 5 min. (increase from baseline respiratory rate >10 breaths/min.), heart rate increase >20%, S$_a$O$_2$ < 90%, patient becomes anxious or diaphoretic.

   v. Return the patient to the original ventilator settings and document findings including RSB and P0.1.

   vi. Notify the physician if the patient is successful at 2 hrs.

b. Respiratory measurements (static weaning criteria) will be taken as needed. Negative inspiratory force, vital capacity, spontaneous respiratory frequency, spontaneous minute volume will be measured and charted.

c. "Wean to spontaneous mode"

   i. Maintain P$_a$O$_2$ and P$_a$CO$_2$ within limits specified in "5, a, b" above

   ii. Maintain patient status within limits specified in "6, a,iv" above

   iii. Reduce F$_I$O$_2$ to 0.4 as indicated

   iv. May change to SIMV mode if necessary and incrementally reduce SIMV to spontaneous mode within 2 hrs.

   v. Reduce PSV to 5 cmH$_2$O

   vi. If the patient tolerates spontaneous ventilation well, then check ABG after 30 min on Spon., PEEP 5, PSV = 5-10 cmH$_2$O. ABG is not necessary if S$_a$O$_2$ and ETCO$_2$ monitoring is adequate.

d. "Wean to extubate"

   i. Procedure is the same as "6,c"

ii. If the patient tolerates spontaneous ventilation, then assess for extubation and extubate if appropriate.

iii. Refer to the extubation policy and procedure.

Quality of Care/ Ventilator Care Quality Improvement

Mechanical ventilation of humans is a risky and highly dangerous activity considering all the possible things that can go wrong and considering the very high mortality rate. There are many aspects of patient safety including, but not limited to, equipment choice, patient monitoring and health of the ICU staff.

It is important that the hospital has a well designed and constructed ICU that is equipped with state-of-the-art ventilators and peripheral equipment. It affects ventilator patient care that highest standards of practice are in place and the ICU staff have up to date education on all aspects of ICU patient care.

With so much needed attention to critical details it matters if the respiratory therapist, ICU nurse or intensivist are having a bad day either at work or bringing in pressures from home. If an ICU team member is ill, taking medications, having conflict with others, or has an attitude, it will affect patient care, as attentiveness and decision making may be diminished.

It makes a difference to the effectiveness of the procedures how the ICU is staffed and the level of their credentials.

The culture of the ICU is important regarding matters like staff morale, the ability to speak up with problems and suggestions.

All of these aspects and more affect the quality of ventilator patient care.

There are no quality measurements for ventilator care other than the ventilator bundles and surveillance for ventilator associated pneumonia. Medical centers gather data and report on various aspects of those processes. Cardiac surgery quality databases require reporting of the length of ventilator stay following certain major cardiac surgeries.

As mentioned above in regard to defining VAE/VAP, there has been a struggle by medicine to measure ventilator days. The struggle is not that it isn't valuable. It is that it is not valued enough to be done correctly.

Ventilator Length of Stay (VLOS) is a potential quality measure for all ventilator patients. VLOS should be measured precisely and reported as ventilator hours which is easily translated to ventilator days by dividing by 24 hrs. in a day. VLOS can be measured easily by noting the time of intubation and placement on the ventilator and the time when the ventilator is weaned or discontinued.

VLOS is an outcome measure and can be correlated with many meaningful aspects of ventilator care like patient age, pulmonary diagnosis, mortality, time of day, day of the week, the physician responsible for the ventilator and other factors that could be chosen by examination of National best practices or specific interests of a particular medical center, ICU, respiratory care department or intensivist group.

It is easy to see that getting patients off the ventilator sooner is a big opportunity to reduce risk and assure better ventilator patient safety. This quality measure has yet to be adopted.

CHAPTER 8

Discontinuation of the Ventilator or "Weaning"

Theories of Weaning

Getting the ventilator patient off the machine can be super easy or extremely difficult or unsuccessful.

The most important concept to getting the patient off the ventilator is answering the question, "Why is this patient on the ventilator?" at least every day, if not every shift or every few hours. Another critical point is keeping them off of the ventilator in the first place, avoiding unnecessary intubation and ventilation by considering options to placing patients on ventilators.

It is reasonable to expect a thorough assessment of the patient at least once a shift by the intensivist, respiratory therapist and ICU nurse. It is best if this can be done together at the first of the shift.

Many ICUs have multidisciplinary rounds at least daily. This is when the ICU team including intensivist, ICU nurses, respiratory therapists, dieticians, pastors, lab technicians, occupational therapy, physical therapy, case management and other interested parties assess and evaluate all aspects of the patient on a ventilator. This allows the ICU team to participate in producing a plan for the day and should improve the patient's chances of survival and getting off the ventilator.

Without this meeting each professional may develop their own plan for the patient for the day or not. This results in a certain amount of chaos or lack of planning and the patient may end up on the ventilator longer than necessary. In practice, sometimes healthcare workers are so focused on all the details of ventilator patient management and some current crisis that they frequently fail to assess and analyze the reason the patient is on the ventilator. This is unfortunate.

The best automated ventilator protocols assess the need for the patient to be on the ventilator breath-to-breath and reduce or increase support as indicated on a real time basis. These automated protocols have been shown to reduce ventilator length of stay.

There are also respiratory therapist driven protocols for ventilator discontinuation that receive a lot of positive attention. (See Chapter 7)

You will see in the discussion below that it is difficult to determine when a patient is ready to breathe on their own, and that it is labor intensive and somewhat risky to conduct a weaning trial.

At this time the best method of ventilator discontinuation for short term ventilator stay, a few hours, is to assess the patient. If ready, take off the ventilator, pull out the endotracheal tube, and let the patient resume normal breathing. The procedure goes like this: The physician ordering the ventilator, typically an anesthesiologist or emergency physician, checks that the patient is awake and responsive, looks to make sure that vital signs are stable, asks the patient to demonstrate a cough, asks the patient if they want the endotracheal tube out. If all is positive, the ventilator is removed, the endotracheal tube is removed, the patient is placed on a minimal amount of oxygen or cool mist and the nursing staff monitor the patient. Everyone lives happily ever after.

The current best method for the longer-term ventilator patient, a day to a few weeks, is the spontaneous breathing trial (SBT) where the patient is removed from all but the most minimal support and allowed to try to breathe on their own. This is usually done every morning after sedation of the patient has been turned off or minimized. If the patient begins to fail, full ventilation and sedation are reapplied. If they succeed, the ventilator will be discontinued. The procedure for SBT is detailed in Chapter 7.

It is my observation that the world-wide success of SBT is proof that the health care team really does not know what they are doing in terms of discontinuing ventilators. If we really knew what we were doing, patients would be discontinued from ventilators at any time in the 24 hr. day, whenever they are ready. The problem is we don't understand well enough when the patient is ready to breathe on their own, so we have to give them a best shot at it every morning. This statement is not meant to demean the ICU team, but to put into perspective the state of the art or rather lack of science regarding ventilator weaning.

Measures of Readiness to Wean

The causes of ventilator dependency are the same factors that cause people to have to go on the ventilator in the first place. To take the patient off the ventilator we must measure the same kinds of things that caused us to put them on the ventilator initially. We assess how well we have reversed the causes of their need for mechanical ventilation. In addition, we assess any newly developed conditions that may have occurred to the patient from having been intubated and on a ventilator.

Recall why the patient cannot move enough air in and out of their lungs by themselves:

1. They cannot get enough oxygen from their lungs into their blood. The percent oxygen and PEEP level they are receiving is still too high.
2. Their airway resistance is too high in either the bronchial tubes or artificial airways
3. Their lung compliance is too low as lungs or chest walls are too stiff.
4. Their breathing muscles are still too weak to get enough tidal volume or respiratory rate.
5. They have increased VD/VT, the blood going to their lungs is not matching with the air being breathed in.
6. Their respiratory stimulus from the brain remains impaired or absent.
7. There may be non-respiratory factors that require mechanical ventilator support such as cardiovascular factors, and psychological dependence.

Before we try a spontaneous breathing trial, we will determine if it is safe for the patient to reduce the oxygen, PEEP and try breathing spontaneously. Ventilator patients with a very high level of support cannot and should not be given SBT.

How do we determine if it is safe to place the patient in a spontaneous breathing trial?

According to 2002 American Association for Respiratory Care Guidelines, printed in the Respiratory Care Journal, we will consider the following criteria to see if patients on high level of mechanical support can tolerate the SBT. These guidelines are technical; however, if you have read this book up to this point, you should be ok. Otherwise, refer to the glossary when needed.

Table 3.   Criteria Used in Weaning/Discontinuation Studies to
           Determine Whether Patients Receiving High Levels of
           Ventilatory Support Can Be Considered for
           Discontinuation (ie, Entered Into the Trials)*

Objective Measurements	Adequate oxygenation (eg, $P_{O_2} \geq 60$ mm Hg on $F_{IO_2} \leq 0.4$; PEEP ≤ 5–10 cm H_2O; $P_{O_2}/F_{IO_2} \geq 150$–300)
	Stable cardiovascular system (eg, HR $\leq$ 140 beats/min; stable blood pressure; no or minimal vasopressors)
	Afebrile (eg, temperature $< 38°C$)
	No significant respiratory acidosis
	Adequate hemoglobin (eg, Hgb ≥ 8–10 g/dL)
	Adequate mentation (eg, arousable, GCS ≥ 13, no continuous sedative infusions
	Stable metabolic status (eg, acceptable electrolytes)
Subjective Clinical Assessments	Resolution of disease acute phase; physician believes discontinuation possible; adequate cough

---

P_{O_2} = partial pressure of oxygen
F_{IO_2} = fraction of inspired oxygen
PEEP = positive end-expiratory pressure
HR = heart rate
GCS = Glasgow Coma Scale
*Adapted from References 101–103, 107–109, 119, and 120

Regarding information in the table above, if the P/F ratio is nearer to 300 or higher, the patient will have a much better chance of weaning.

In addition, there are other clinical measurements that are sometimes considered.

NIF (negative inspiratory force) or how hard can the patient suck in a breath when asked to try very hard. This should be at least -20 to -30 cmH$_2$O.

IVC (inspiratory vital capacity) or how large a volume of air can the patient breathe in when asked to try very hard. This should be more than 10 ml/Kg body weight.

NIF and IVC have been used for a long time. Although they seem like good measures, they do not correlate very well with successful breathing and extubation.

If the patient is breathing spontaneously on the ventilator the following measures may be considered.

RSBI (Rapid Shallow Breathing Index) or the respiratory rate divided by the tidal volume (f/TV). This should be more than 105. This value correlates well (70 - 80%) with successful spontaneous breathing. Basically, it is a number that represents that the patient is not breathing too fast (f) nor too shallowly (TV) to be able to breathe on their own. Kind of common sense if you can't breathe in a decent tidal volume and are huffing and puffing rapidly, chances are you are not going to last long breathing on your own.

P0.1 (Inspiratory Pressure within the first 1/10 sec.) This should not be more than 3 - 5 cmH_2O. This can only be measured on a microprocessor-controlled ventilator. Simplified, it is a number that reflects if a patient is gasping for a breath or breathing quietly. P0.1 correlates well (about 70%) with successful ventilator discontinuation. Once again, common sense, if the patient is gasping for air it is not likely they are ready to get off the ventilator.

f (respiratory rate or breaths per minute) This should be less than 30/min. When people have to breathe over 30 breaths/minute they usually fail SBT. If you see someone who is not exercising breathing this fast, probably better keep an eye on them and make sure your phone is charged.

Minute volume (volume of air breathed in and out in a minute) This should be less than 10 - 15 liters/minute. If the patient is breathing more than this, they will tire out or they have increased deadspace ventilation and likely fail SBT.

Finally, there are qualitative measures like having an adequate cough, being cooperative, and ability to lift their head off the pillow. Another qualitative measure that has been studied and highly correlates with successful SBT is just "ask the ICU nurse." If the ICU nurse says the patient is ready for ventilator discontinuation, it is very likely true.

Spontaneous Breathing Trial Protocol

SBT is discussed in Chapter 7. as it is the national and international standard of practice.

IMV Weaning

Intermittent Mandatory Ventilation (IMV) is actually a mode of ventilation that allows patients to breathe spontaneously while on the ventilator. It was first used on the BabyBird ventilator in the early 1970s and saved the lives of hundreds of thousands of newborn babies. In its original form the IMV, intermittent mechanical breath, just slammed into the patient without regard to the patient's breathing cycle. It just delivered the mandatory breath at a certain time when the patient may have been breathing in or breathing out or mid-breath. IMV in current times is called SIMV because the periodic mandatory breaths from the ventilator are synchronized with the patient's effort and dovetail in with the initiation of the patient's own breath.

IMV or SIMV weaning is simply slowly turning down the number of mandatory mechanical breaths given by the ventilator until it is very low or turned off, and the patient is breathing spontaneously. Spontaneous breathing in SIMV can be boosted by pressure support during the inspiratory phase allowing the patient to take a bigger breath. This pressure support must be reduced during IMV weaning, so the patient is actually doing most of the work to breathe. Otherwise, they will fail weaning.

IMV weaning is not a commonly used method because studies have shown it to be less effective than SBT. It is interesting that weaning by automated ventilators is done by IMV weaning and pressure support weaning quite successfully. It may be that artificial intelligence is paying better attention to the patient than the human ICU team.

Pressure Support Weaning

Spontaneous breathing can be boosted by pressure support during the inspiratory phase allowing the patient to take a bigger breath. The patient starts taking a breath and the machine slides in some positive pressure to give the patient a little more volume. Actually, pressure support can give quite a bit more volume if it is set high enough.

During pressure support weaning the patient could be placed on spontaneous mode breathing with a relatively high-pressure support. Then pressure support will be incrementally reduced so the patient is actually doing most of the work to breathe.

Pressure support weaning is not a commonly used method because studies have shown it to be less effective than SBT. Again, it is interesting that weaning by automated ventilators is done by IMV and pressure support weaning.

Automated Ventilator Weaning

There are a number of very complex ways automated ventilators assess the patient's need for mechanical ventilation and provide the patient enough support by increasing pressures, volumes, respiratory rate and a number of other factors. ASV, AVM, NAVA, and SmartCare+ are all among proprietary names for ventilator modes that include, or are designed for, ventilator weaning.

Perhaps a word about the acronyms. Adaptive Support Ventilation (ASV) is a Hamilton Medical product that is joined with Intellicare to be the most sophisticated automated ventilator modality in the world. Unfortunately, its automated, closed-loop oxygen and PEEP functions are not available in the USA. ASV monitors minute volume, tidal volume, expiratory resistance, lung/thorax compliance, frequency of control breaths, frequency of spontaneous breaths, and peak inspiratory pressure. As a result, the ventilator computer knows if the patient is breathing and how much; as well as knowing the airway resistance and lung/thoracic compliance which it includes in how much support the patient will need. It does this breath-to-breath and makes breath-to-breath changes while looking back at the previous three breaths. The ventilator computer automatically changes mode of ventilation, inspiratory pressure, inspiratory time, and respiratory frequency. As a result, the ventilator length of stay (LOS) is lower, and the patient appears more comfortable.

Adaptive Ventilation Mode on the Bella Vista 1000 ventilator by Vyaire is similar to ASV, and adds "auto rise, "auto leak" and "auto sync" functionality that should make the patient more comfortable. It does not close-the-loop on oxygen and PEEP.

Neurally Adjusted Ventilatory Assist (NAVA) SERVO-i ventilator by Getinge can be used with their Automode making an automated mode of ventilation that is super sensitive and is advertised for weaning. Electrical activity of the diaphragm (Edi) is captured from a probe that goes down the esophagus and sends a signal to the ventilator computer to assist the patient's breathing in synchrony with and in proportion to the patient's own efforts. As the work of the ventilator and the diaphragm is controlled by the same signal, the coupling between the diaphragm and the ventilator is synchronized simultaneously.

SmartCare PS by Draeger on the Evita ventilator is an automated clinical protocol, designed to stabilize the patient's spontaneous breathing in a comfortable zone of normal ventilation and to automatically reduce the ventilatory support thereby weaning the patient from the ventilator. SmartCare monitors respiratory rate, tidal volume and end-tidal CO_2; then it changes the pressure support appropriately.

Since the automated ventilator is assessing the patient's needs every breath or very frequently, it calculates when the patient is ready to receive more or less support constantly. If it determines the patient needs less support, it has algorithms that safely wean the patient to spontaneous breathing. Then the patient is ready for ventilator discontinuation. The automated ventilator protocol has extensive monitoring and safety systems in place during the process and storage of the monitored data. There is no need for SBT unless the ICU ventilator team is being very cautious. To keep the patient safe during weaning these automated protocols will also give more ventilatory support if the patient becomes weaker.

The adoption of automated ventilation has been slow among intensivists. It is difficult to determine why use of automated ventilation has been taking off slowly. Some reasons are surely that many ventilators don't yet have automation, all automated protocols are not similarly effective, and physicians are slow to change because lives depend on their decisions.

T-Piece Weaning

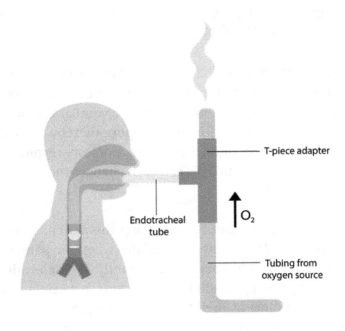

Illustration of a T-piece Weaning Set-up

T-piece weaning is one of the oldest methods of weaning and is still used; even though studies have shown it to be less effective than SBT. T-piece weaning is potentially the most dangerous weaning procedure as the patient is removed from the ventilator and placed on a T-piece adapter hooked up to an oxygenated mist without any mechanical support. T-piece weaning is carefully monitored with the respiratory therapist or nurse physically present during the first 10 - 20 mins. Please see the setup diagrammed on the previous page. The problem with T-piece weaning is that it takes the patient from nearly full ventilator support to almost nothing with the hope that the patient did not need the ventilator. Even though the patient is closely monitored by the respiratory therapist and nurse there may be lasting consequences if the patient fails the T-piece trial. Those consequences could include some lung collapse from no PEEP, acidosis from hypoxia and hypercapnia, any side-effects from cardiac stress, and anxiety produced by failure.

Miscellaneous Weaning Methods

There is a myriad of weaning methods practiced by various pulmonary physicians and intensivists. Most of these methods are poorly studied and their merit has not been established. The important thing is that the patient is monitored closely and not placed in jeopardy.

Weaning chronic ventilator patients who have been on the ventilator for months or years is not the subject of this book.

Criteria for Weaning Trial Failure

Patients frequently succeed and often fail weaning trials. They could get into serious breathing or cardiac problems if not monitored closely. Weaning trial failure looks about the same regardless of the method.

We will look at criteria for SBT success. If the numbers or observations are worse than those below, the SBT is stopped and the patient is returned to the previous ventilator settings.

SBT criteria include acceptable levels of oxygen as S_pO_2 greater than 85 to 90%; P_aO_2 greater than 50 - 60 mmHg; pH greater than 7.32; and increase in P_aCO_2 less than 10 mmHg. These criteria show that the patient is getting enough oxygen and the carbon dioxide is not building up excessively.

SBT criteria for hemodynamic stability should include a heart rate less than 120 beats per minute and not have changed more than 20%. Blood pressure must remain between 180/90 mmHg and not have changed more than 20% without vasopressor drugs being required. These criteria show the heart is getting enough oxygen and is able to do its work without help from drugs or too much stress.

Subjective assessment of SBT includes any change in mental status including becoming too sleepy, going into a coma, agitation, anxiety, and combativeness. If the patient feels uncomfortable and complains of shortness of breath and dyspnea (difficulty breathing) it may be time to go back on the ventilator. If the patient breaks out in a sweat (diaphoresis) or has signs of increased work of breathing like struggling and/or using accessory muscles of breathing, it is a sign of failure.

It is considered a success if the patient can tolerate the SBT well for 30 mins to 2 hours. In that case the ventilator will be discontinued.

Extubation

Extubation, removing the endotracheal tube, is a different question than removing the ventilator. Extubation decision is made on the ability of the patient to maintain a natural airway (airway patency) and ability to keep their airways clear of obstruction, especially mucus.

Airway patency may have been compromised by traumatic intubation attempts or irritation of the airway by the tracheal tube or its balloon that seals against the tender wall of the trachea. Before extubation the respiratory therapist must deflate the tracheal tube balloon and ascertain if there is room for air movement around the tube. If the patient's trachea is swollen up against the tube, the patient will not be able to breathe after removing the tube. A bad outcome.

Ability to keep the airway open is also a matter of having a strong enough cough and being cooperative enough to cough when asked.

Follow Up Care

Former ventilator patients must be watched closely after ventilator discontinuation and extubation. Every effort must be made to help them maintain spontaneous breathing and prevent future collapse and return to the ventilator. It is a serious oversight to not pay enough attention to a recently weaned and extubated patient and allow them to decompensate and end up back on the ventilator.

Patients weaned from ventilators may be immediately transferred to step-down ICU or a Telemetry Unit. They will remain in ICU if they have other serious ICU level issues.

CHAPTER 9

Diseases That May Require Mechanical Ventilation

This chapter will allow the reader to see how different disease entities present different challenges or even, perhaps, make the use of the ventilator easier. We will first look at what should be relatively easy cases before jumping into extremely difficult COVID-19 and its associated ARDS.

Post-op Cardiac and Other Major Surgery

Some operative procedures require mechanical ventilation during recovery from surgery for a few hours or overnight. This may be due to the need for continued paralysis and/or sedation. It may be due to the complexity of the surgery like liver, lung, and heart transplants. Mechanical ventilation is sometimes part of the cardiac surgeon's post-operative recovery protocol for open heart surgery patients who are then extubated several hours later or the morning after surgery.

In most of these cases these patients have normal lungs and are waiting for sedation to wear off, to be discontinued, or the patient is being supported overnight for the surgery effects to stabilize.

These patients are maintained on minimal amounts of oxygen (30 - 40%) and PEEP (5-8 cmH$_2$O), so that when the ICU team is ready to discontinue the ventilator in a few hours or in the morning, the patient is awakened, assessed, the ventilator taken off, and the endotracheal tube removed. Usually a spontaneous breathing trial (SBT) is not necessary.

Bronchial Asthma Exacerbation (Attack)

A severe asthma exacerbation requiring mechanical ventilation actually has a name, "near-fatal asthma". If the patient did not get to the emergency room in time, they would surely have died. In these cases, normal ventilation is compromised by the obstruction of the patient's natural airways by inflammation (swelling) of the walls of the bronchial tube, bronchial muscle spasm (airway constriction) and thick mucus. They are very hard to ventilate due to expiratory and inspiratory airway resistance. Air is trapped deep in their lungs behind these swollen airways on arrival to the Emergency Room, and they cannot exhale, in spite of feeling they can't get their breath in.

Typically, they must be sedated and perhaps paralyzed just before intubation and placement on a ventilator. The "medical coma" may be maintained to better control the airway and ventilation. These patients are very anxious and very tired of struggling to breathe. The ventilator needs to be set carefully to allow more time for exhalation and to avoid very high peak inspiratory pressures. The patient will have already been given bronchodilators to reduce airway muscle constriction, and oral or IV corticosteroids to reduce inflammation on admission to the ER. Usually, the bronchodilators won't help much because the patient was already taking maximum amounts of rescue inhaler bronchodilators at home or pre-admission. These patients may have been on corticosteroids as controller medications at home, so the corticosteroids may not work well either.

This is ventilatory failure, so high oxygen and high PEEP may not be necessary. We just have to ventilate the air in and out to keep the blood carbon dioxide level down. Not an easy task under these circumstances.

In extreme cases it is so difficult to ventilate the near-fatal asthma patient that air is replaced with a helium and oxygen mixture, maybe 20 - 40% oxygen and the remainder helium. Helium is much less dense than nitrogen, the major component of air, and has a better chance of getting in and out of narrow airways as a carrier for oxygen.

In most asthma cases after an overnight stay in ICU on a ventilator, the airway restriction and airway resistance can be reversed. The patient can be extubated in the morning. Once the airway narrowing is reversed the asthma patient can be allowed to wake up and be ventilated in a mode with spontaneous breathing, then the ventilator discontinued.

In the unlikely circumstance that the extreme asthma exacerbation cannot be reversed so soon these patients are some of the most difficult to manage on the ventilator. They require long inspiratory times to avoid high pressures that cause lung injury, and they require long expiratory times to be able to avoid air trapping, auto-PEEP and pneumothorax. With both inspiration and expiration being long the respiratory rate ends up being as low as possible to prevent carbon dioxide build up and development of respiratory acidosis caused by high carbonic acid in the blood. Fortunately, most asthma ventilator patients do well.

Drug Overdose

Overdose from opiate or sedative drugs or other medications may cause the brain to send inadequate or no messages to the respiratory muscles to contract for breathing. This is ventilatory failure. If these patients can be intubated and ventilated very soon, they are very easy to manage on the ventilator. They have normal lungs.

Most of the time after the drug effects have been reversed the ventilated patient can be extubated and the ventilator discontinued. These patients do very well with very high survival.

In the worst-case scenario, which is not infrequent, the overdose patient is not found by someone immediately or did not arrive in the emergency room soon enough. They became unconscious and/or quit breathing prior to being intubated and ventilated. This has two dreadful possibilities:

1. When the patient stops breathing, they have about four to six minutes before their brain and heart tissue start dying. Chances are they will be found dead. If they are found alive, they may be brain dead or partially brain dead when placed on the ventilator. This becomes a very tragic

outcome and makes difficult problems for the patient, loved ones and society in general.

2. When the opiate overdose patient is becoming unconscious and found at that time, they will often lose control of their airway and throw up. The vomit in their mouth and nose pours into their lungs or gets sucked back into their lungs because they have no cough reflexes and may still be breathing. These very acidic gastric contents are extremely damaging to the lungs and easily cause adult acute respiratory distress syndrome (ARDS). ARDS is discussed in detail below.

ARDS with Emphasis on COVID-19

The SARS-COV-2 pandemic is what stimulated the development of this book to help families and friends of victims to understand ventilators and answer questions that come to mind when a loved one is on one of these machines. ARDS is caused by many diverse problems as well as COVID-19. A short list includes pneumonia, near drowning, sepsis, trauma, pulmonary edema, aspiration of gastric contents, inhalation of smoke and hazardous gases.

ARDS may be the most difficult condition faced by ventilator patients and their ICU caregivers. ARDS is primarily oxygenation failure and often becomes severe oxygenation failure caused by disruption of the alveolocapillary membranes deep in the lungs. This disruption causes collapse of the alveoli and actual tearing apart the cells of the membrane. This damaged lung tissue can also slow the excretion of carbon dioxide, so ARDS becomes ventilatory failure on top of oxygenation failure. Ventilatory failure is also caused by decreased lung compliance as the lungs become stiff and "beefy" accompanied by the development of deadspace ventilation, wasted ventilation. In the diagram below, even though there is much more information that we need, these changes can be seen in the very different pictures of normal vs ARDS lung. The micrographs below show the same thing. In the ARDS lung tissue photo the alveolar and capillary walls are all torn apart and fluids are gathering in the air sacs compared to the reasonably well-organized normal slice of lung tissue.

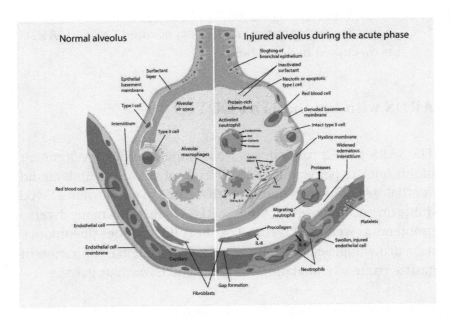

Diagram of Normal and ARDS lung tissue

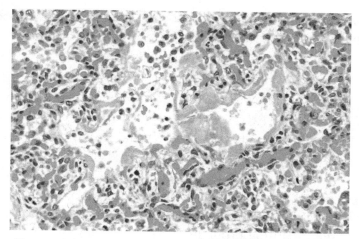

Electron Micrograph of Disorganized ARDS Alveolar Membranes

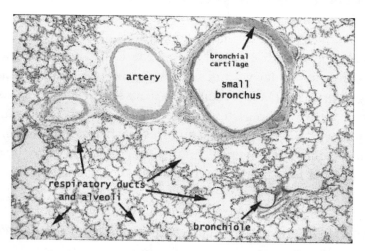

Electron Micrograph of Normal Alveolar Membranes

ARDS is often fatal and survival has not significantly improved since the 1970s. Generally, ARDS survival rate is 50 - 75% of the cases. There are Spring 2020 reports from New York City COVID-19 ARDS ventilator patients declaring a 90% fatality rate. During the same time dismal reports COVID-19 ARDS ventilator patients from China are showing 20 - 40% survival. Survival has to do with multiple factors which include how sick the patient was in the first place, quality of ventilator care, hospital and caregiver resources, co-morbidities (other diseases present) and a range of other complex factors.

Why should a patient even want to go on a ventilator with COVID-19 induced ARDS? Because they want to live!! They will die without the ventilator. A 10 - 40% chance of living is much better than zero.

ARDS is usually managed according to the ARDSNet protocol covered in Chapter 7. In overview the ARDSNet protocol includes defining the breathing problem as ARDS, recommending initial ventilator settings such as tidal volume, oxygen and PEEP levels. ARDSNet directs increasing and decreasing the oxygen and PEEP as necessary, trying to keep the inhaled oxygen as low as reasonably possible and keeping the PEEP, peak inspiratory pressures, and tidal volumes from causing Ventilator Induced Lung Injury (VILI). VILI seems to be caused by excessive positive pressure (barotrauma), excessive lung volumes (volutrauma) and damage to delicate lung structures by sheer forces associated with stretching and over distending lung units that may be over full and abut lung units that are collapsed or partially full.

There is an emerging attention to a condition associated with ARDS called Patient Self-Induced Lung Injury (PS-ILI). Although unclear, this may be caused by spontaneous breathing efforts at smaller lung volumes, lower PEEP, and asynchronous breathing with the ventilator. Amid the COVID-19/ARDS reports there is one suggesting better outcomes with larger tidal volumes and higher PEEP. This information causes this author to speculate that perhaps a few ARDS studies with high ARDS survival (60 - 80%) in the 1970s may have been the best way to ventilate ARDS patients with high tidal volumes, high PEEP and spontaneous breathing. The problem with that approach is keeping VILI minimized, and that the intensivists and respiratory therapists have to perform at a very high level that has seldom been seen since.

Other than the ARDSNet protocol there are other methods of managing ARDS including the use of Airway Pressure Relief Ventilation (APRV) and similar dual pressure modes. Also, the use of automated breathing protocols like Adaptive Support Ventilation or "Intellicare" (Hamilton Medical) have been well studied and manage the ARDS patient according to protocols embedded in the high-end microprocessor-controlled ventilator. Comprehensive ventilator automation called Adaptive Ventilation Mode, (Vyaire Medical) is very similar.

Adjuncts to ARDS ventilator management may include lung recruitment maneuvers, see Chapter 7, permissive hypercapnia, prone positioning, careful management of the patient's fluid balance, a numerous assortment of medications, and some other not well studied techniques.

ARDS causes the ICU team to "try everything and anything", because before the ARDS ventilator patient dies their blood oxygen is dropping in the face of 100% oxygen and highest PEEP, and their carbon dioxide level is rising in face of maximum pressures and respirator rates. At this point the intensivist must talk to the family about futility of care, and possibility of end of life.

This desperation can go so far as to place the patient on an Extracorporeal Membrane Oxygenator (ECMO). ECMO pumps blood that would go to the lungs out of the body through tubes placed in major blood vessels and pumps that deoxygenated blood through an artificial lung where it exchanges carbon dioxide and oxygen. This freshly oxygenated blood is then pumped back into the patient's body and supports their life while their lungs heal themselves. ECMO type machines are frequently and successfully used in cardiac surgery for short periods of time. ECMO results are poor enough with ARDS that there is no clear recommendation to try it or not. Beyond that, many smaller medical centers don't have ECMO equipment or service. In all fairness, it may be that ECMO is often a "last ditch" effort with failing ARDS patients; therefore, does not have much chance of success.

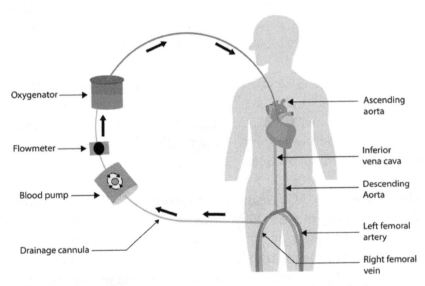

Illustration of an Extracorporeal Membrane Oxygenator hooked up to a patient

The ventilator patient with ARDS can be expected to be on the ventilator for many days to a few weeks. Reports from China stated the COVID-19 ARDS patients were on the ventilator 14 - 21 days. Generally, most ARDS patients will be on the ventilator for one to three weeks or more. When they come off the ventilator alive, they have to participate in serious physical rehabilitation.

This discussion of the management of ARDS patients is overly simplified as it focuses on just the ventilator. In fact, while struggling with all the ventilator factors, the intensivist and ICU nurses are working to maintain stability of the patient's heart, kidneys, mental status, nutrition, skin integrity, fluid and electrolyte balance, and about anything else that can go wrong.

Heart Attack

Mechanical ventilation may be needed as a result of heart attack.

Hopefully in these days of prevention and public awareness heart attacks can be avoided or at least recognized early and treated early and effectively without the need of mechanical ventilators. Heart and blood vessel disease is the #1 cause of death of people in the USA.

Mechanical ventilators are often needed if a heart attack victim survives cardiopulmonary resuscitation (CPR). A few CPR survivors may have little or no damage to the lungs and not need a ventilator. They can be treated like any other heart disease patient.

Many CPR survivors have some serious breathing problems following resuscitation. They may have lung contusion (bruising), broken ribs, lung laceration, pneumothorax (holes between the lung and the pleura), left heart failure which backs up blood and pressure which pushes fluid back into the lungs, brain death and other organ death, laceration of the diaphragm, traumatic intubation, and aspiration of gastric contents among other things. Each of these problems will need to be handled differently. It may be the ARDSNet protocol, above. It may be pneumothorax/bronchopleural fistula, below. It may be a brain injury. The CPR survivor may have multi-organ failure (heart, lungs, kidneys, brain, liver). This is a real challenge to the intensivist and ICU team.

Obesity

When people get morbidly obese and their weight gets over 450 - 750 lbs, they can experience ventilatory failure and will die if not placed on a ventilator. This ventilatory failure is caused by decreased chest wall compliance. The abdominal weight fatigues the diaphragm and muscles of respiration, weight on the chest makes it further difficult to breathe and fatty tissues around the upper airways cause obstruction to breathing.

The ventilator management of these patients is simple as they have normal lungs. We let the ventilator do the work of breathing, and the tracheal tube will hold the airway open. The big problem is reversing the underlying problem, obesity. It takes a long time, and it is dangerous to lose a few hundred pounds. In addition, every other aspect of managing these large patients is very difficult. They require special beds, special nutrition, extra personnel to turn, bathe and do patient care. They will likely be on the ventilator for months and require a tracheostomy. If the healthcare team can prevent injury and stupid mistakes during this long time, these patients will do very well.

Neurosurgery, Brain Trauma, Stroke and Intracranial Bleeding

Ventilation of patients with head trauma whether from injury, surgery or stroke are easy because their lungs are normal. Low levels of oxygen and PEEP can maintain brain trauma patients with normal tidal volumes and respiratory rate. Pressure in the brain must be kept low or normal. One consideration is that high pressures in the chest caused by the positive pressure ventilation must be avoided because those pressures will be partially transmitted to the brain. Secondly, carbon dioxide is a cerebral vasodilator (opens up blood flow and pressure to the brain). Carbon dioxide must be managed intelligently to keep it at normal P_aCO_2 = 35 - 45 mmHg or less.

The final consideration is that of the patient waking up and whether or not they are able to breathe. Perhaps parts of the brain controlling respirations may have been permanently damaged. If there is irreparable damage to the patient's ability to breath, and they are awake and responsive; they may spend the rest of their life on a ventilator. That sounds horrible, but with good long-term ventilator care the patient can establish a new, compromised quality of life and be happy for many years. On the other hand, if the patient is miserable and can't get beyond that, it is an extremely difficult way to live. The other possibility is that the patient doesn't wake up at all and is in a permanent coma. It may even be determined that they are brain dead.

Vegetative life with brain death on a ventilator, tube feeding and other life support without any quality of life is a dismal situation. Most of us would not want to exist like this. That is why we often hear people say, "I don't want life support, just unplug me." After reading this far you can see this is probably not a wise statement;

because much of the time people survive ventilators with high quality of life, and if the ventilator is unplugged the battery backup will kick in and keep the ventilator running.

It is important to note that brain death determination must be done according to medical and legal protocol. Mistakes in this determination are intolerable. How to deal with brain dead patients on ventilators is a perfect example of an instance where technology (life support) has advanced beyond social, religious and psychological mechanisms to deal with it. There have been a number of famous cases in the news on this subject with the family wanting life support left on or taken off and the medical center wanting to do the opposite and it all ends up in court.

Neuromuscular Disease

Neuromuscular diseases like amyotrophic lateral sclerosis (ALS), muscular dystrophy, Guillian-Barre Syndrome and others may lead the patient to a slow decline into ventilatory failure. As their muscles become weaker, they are just not strong enough to breathe, and the P_aCO_2 rises. After every other intervention is tried, these patients may end up on a ventilator. It is likely, not certain, to be long term, or perhaps, the rest of their life. They are easy to ventilate because they have essentially normal lungs. They are difficult patients; because it is so heartbreaking to be involved in their neuromuscular decline and placement on mechanical ventilation when they are fully awake and cognizant. This requires a lot of involvement of case management, family, friends, and perhaps pastoral care. Another possible example of "it takes a village."

Trauma/Injury

Several forms of injury can result in the use of mechanical ventilators. Clearly, chest trauma like getting the chest crushed in a car crash or penetrated by gunshot or stabbing in the chest and lung. The number of possible causes is too large to list.

Mechanical ventilation of these patients is varied depending on the extent of injury and what anatomy is affected. These injuries may have a relatively simple surgical solution to sew up the wounds or may be dreadful injury breaking ribs, puncturing the lungs, diaphragm, heart and major blood vessels and major loss of blood. These patients may be treated as ARDS (above) or pneumothorax/bronchopleural fistula (below).

Other trauma affecting the lungs are those that create pulmonary embolism like long bone fracture producing fatty embolism (fat blobs) that float to the lungs, large vein trauma or decompression injury (scuba diving errors) producing air embolism. These pulmonary emboli clog up the blood flow to the lungs causing areas of the lungs to be without blood flow but are being ventilated. We know it as dead space or wasted ventilation. This can be just enough to need mechanical ventilation or may be fatal within minutes. The resolution is stopping the emboli and reversing the emboli already in the lungs.

Near-Drowning

Everybody knows "drowning" is the term for those who die under water. Near-drowning is a term for those who survive the struggle against drowning. Hopefully, most people who nearly drown are rescued without many consequences as they don't get water down in their lungs nor quit breathing. They may get checked out by a doctor or not.

The ventilator management of near-drowning is usually ARDS for those who get much water into their lungs.

Fresh water near-drowning allows fresh water in the lungs that has no or little salt. This water is pulled across the alveolocapillary membrane from the lungs into the blood very rapidly. Thus, destroying the integrity of the alveolocapillary membrane which results in ARDS. The fresh water may also contain contaminants of various kinds like mud, sewage, chlorine, etc. Each contaminant adds its additional problems to the lung tissue. In this situation the blood volume may become too large and diluted, or even the red blood cells can swell with fresh water and rupture which adds additional problems.

Salt water in the lungs is just the opposite, having more salt than the blood. Saltwater in the lungs pulls water from the blood across the alveolocapillary membrane into the lungs, destroying its integrity and resulting in ARDS. In this situation the lungs are full of fluid. The blood volume may become too low and concentrated which adds additional problems.

Either way the near-drowning patient with ARDS is challenging to mechanically ventilate.

Pneumothorax/Bronchopleural fistula

Pneumothorax (pneumo [air] in the thorax [chest cavity]) can come from a punctured lung where air from inside the lung can get in between the lung and the chest wall creating a pocket of air. Please see the diagram below. This can be relatively minor requiring only a chest drainage tube (a tube inserted through the skin between the ribs) from the outside to let the air out. The chest tube is usually connected to a sealed container to collect the air or any fluids that might be coming out of the patient's pleural space. The images below illustrate pneumothorax and its treatment with a chest tube and drainage system.

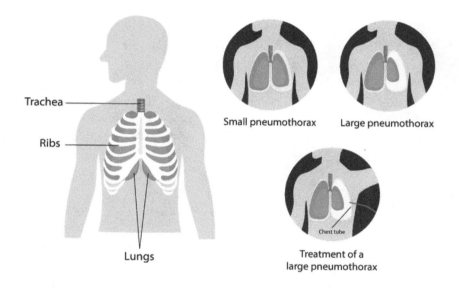

Pneumothorax illustration with different size "Pneumos"

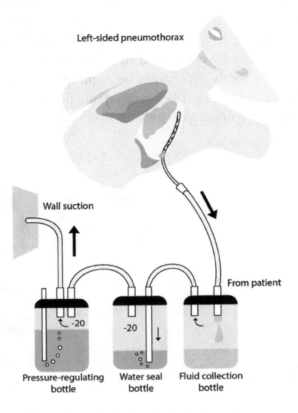

Illustration of a chest tube drainage system

Pneumothorax can happen to a few people spontaneously, meaning it can happen at any time. It is best not to use a ventilator in these cases as the positive pressure ventilator can make the pneumothorax worse by pushing air out the hole in the lung, making pneumothorax bigger and the lung smaller. Sometimes the pneumothorax can be caused by the ventilator rupturing lung tissue, VILI. The ICU team must assess the resolution of the pneumothorax. If the ventilator starts pumping air into the pneumothorax cavity, and it goes out the chest tube in any measurable volume, this is called a bronchopleural fistula, a hole through the lung and the pleura to the outside of the body. Bronchopleural fistula (BP fistula) is a very unfortunate development, and its resolution (getting closed up) is a high priority. Resolution of BP fistula is beyond this discussion.

Ventilator management in this condition is focused on keeping the pressures as low as possible and assessment of the amount of tidal volume going into the patient with respect to the amount going through the BP fistula to the chest tube system. Clearly the tidal volume going out the hole in the chest is not doing the patient any good for oxygenation or ventilation.

Chronic Obstructive Pulmonary Disease (COPD)

COPD is two similar diseases, pulmonary emphysema and chronic bronchitis. COPD obstructs the bronchial tubes and alveoli (air sacs) by the tissue becoming fibrotic. Fibrosis can cause the bronchial tubes and alveoli to thicken and/or collapse. In chronic bronchitis the bronchial tubes are also inflamed and producing too much thick mucus.

The advanced COPD patient is primarily suffering from ventilatory failure and oxygenation failure is secondary. We try to avoid placing COPD patients on ventilators because there is little or no ability to reverse the underlying condition and so they might be "stuck" on the ventilator. It is very important for advanced COPD patients to have end of life conversations with their physicians, so everyone knows what the patient wants (see Chapter 1, advanced directives and POLST).

Acute exacerbation of COPD can be caused by pneumonia. In this case the underlying cause can be reversed, and the ventilator discontinued after a few days.

Each time a COPD patient succumbs to pneumonia and needs a ventilator, the patient ends up a little worse off. By the third intubation it is most likely the patient will become a chronic ventilator patient. Few people want to live like that; however, some people might choose to stay on a ventilator. In these cases, the patient, their social support system, and a team from the medical center have to figure out whether the patient can go home with a ventilator or to a long-term ventilator facility.

Pneumonia (bacterial, viral, fungal)

Pneumonia is an infection of the lungs from bacteria, virus or other germs that can be acquired at home or in the hospital. It may first seem like a common cold or flu, and then the patient starts having severe problems breathing. It is thought COVID-19 is a viral pneumonia. Pneumonia can develop into ARDS. The goal is to reverse the infection. This is easier with bacteria as bacteria may be killed by antibiotics. Unfortunately, viruses are not killed by antibiotics. For example, as of Fall 2020 we have no effective treatment for COVID-19. There are few medicines effective against fungal infections. In these cases, we have to give the patients medicines that can help their immune system fight the infections and keep the patient alive in the meantime. The outcome for ventilator patients with pneumonia are much better if ARDS does not develop. If it does develop into ARDS the outcome is less than 60% survival like ARDS. The goal for mechanical ventilation of pneumonia patients is life support until the pneumonia can be reversed. When pneumonia is this bad it can result in some permanent lung damage.

Glossary of Terms

Absorption Atelectasis - alveolar collapse secondary to the washout of nitrogen, an inert gas that normally helps maintain alveolar volume

Adjuncts to CMV – PEEP, CPAP, IPAP, EPAP, PCV, VCV, and PSV

Advanced Directive - specifies consent or refuse consent to any care, treatment, service, or procedure to maintain, diagnose, or otherwise affect a physical or mental condition. Advanced Directives may designate specific health-care providers and institutions, desire for organ donation; as well as, address approval or disapproval of diagnostic tests, surgical procedures, programs of medication, orders not to resuscitate; giving artificial nutrition and hydration

Afebrile - no fever, 37 degrees C. or 98.6 degrees F

Alveolocapillary membrane - is actually two very thin membranes; the alveolar membrane up against the pulmonary capillary membrane. They are very delicate, highly efficient, and easily damaged

Alveolar deadspace - is abnormal because it should have blood flow and exchange oxygen and carbon dioxide

Alveolus - is a microscopic air sac that allows rapid exchange of oxygen and carbon dioxide with the blood through its thin membrane (about 0.1 microns thick) and the thin blood capillary membrane

Ambu bag - Ambu is a brand name of a manufacturer of manual resuscitation bags or bag/valve/mask resuscitators. It is used commonly like the words, Kleenex or Xerox copy.

Anatomic deadspace - normal airways that don't exchange gases like the trachea and bronchi

Anoxia - means absence of oxygen, or nearly absent oxygen. Anoxic brain injury is caused by lack of oxygen supply to the brain for more than 4 - 6 minutes

ΔP – peak inspiratory pressure minus baseline pressure, this pressure change from baseline to peak will give the patient a mechanical breath. Air moves on a pressure gradient.

Apnea - absence of breathing. Usually, ventilators alarm and back-up a patient after 20 secs. of apnea. Apnea is defined by a shorter time in a sleep lab

Apnea back-up mode - is a preset respiratory rate and tidal volume on the ventilator that will automatically start breathing the patient after 20 secs. of apnea

APRV - airway pressure relief ventilation is a mode of ventilation where the ventilator holds the patient at a P_{high} for a period of time, T_{high}, and periodically drops the pressure to a P_{low} for a set time T_{low}. P_{low} is about the same as PEEP. The change in pressure (ΔP) during the pressure drop is exhalation. The ventilator then returns to P_{high}. This ΔP during the pressure increase is added benefit of the patient being able to breathe at P_{high} and at P_{low}.

ARDS - can be caused by COVID-19, "Acute Respiratory Distress Syndrome is an acute diffuse, inflammatory lung injury, leading to increased pulmonary vascular permeability, increased lung weight, and loss of aerated lung tissue...[with] hypoxemia and bilateral radiographic opacities, associated with increased venous admixture, increased physiological dead space and decreased lung compliance." 2012 Berlin Definition. Radiographic opacities are evidence of wet or collapsed areas of the lungs. Venous admixture is referring to R-L intrapulmonary shunt (decreased P/F ratio)

Arteries - are blood vessels that take fresh oxygenated blood out to all parts of the body. When we feel a pulse, we are feeling an artery pulsating from the heart pumping

Arterial blood gases or "blood gases" - a lab test to check how much oxygen and carbon dioxide are in the blood. This is the best test result to check the patient's breathing and use of the ventilator as this blood just came through the heart unchanged from the lungs

Aspiration - inhalation of some foreign material; aspiration of vomitus, blood, or mucus may occur when a person is unconscious. When a person is conscious it usually causes choking

Aspiration - withdrawal of fluid by an aspirator; the method is widely used in hospitals. Aspirators may be suction catheters, syringes or other devices

Assist-control mode - this is a ventilator mode of breathing where the operator sets the ventilator to give the same size, type and rate of breathing every breath. If the patient wants an additional breath of the same size and type, when they try to breathe in the sensitive ventilator will supply that breath

Atelectasis - a collapsed or airless state of the lung, which may be acute or chronic, and may involve all or part of the lung

Atelectrauma - lung injury caused by high shear forces from cyclic opening and collapse of atelectatic, but recruitable lung units. Alveolus that are going from collapsed to partially open may generate these shear forces

Barotrauma - pulmonary barotrauma from invasive mechanical ventilation refers to alveolar rupture due to elevated transpulmonary pressure; air leaks into extra-alveolar tissue resulting in conditions including pneumothorax

BiPAP - bi-level positive airway pressure is a trademark of the Respironics Company, it is commonly used to refer to non-invasive ventilation (NIV) and includes IPAP and EPAP. BiPAP is a mechanical ventilator connected to the patient with a face mask instead of a tracheal tube

Bronchi - are large airway tubes that branch off the bottom of the windpipe (trachea) into the right and left lung, bronchi have cartilage supporting the walls of the tube. The bronchi continue to branch smaller and smaller until they have muscular walls and no cartilage. At this point they are called bronchioles

Bronchioles - these smaller airways do not have cartilage or mucus-secreting goblet cells. They have muscular walls and club cells that produce a surfactant lipoprotein which is instrumental in preventing the walls of the small airways sticking together during expiration

C_aO_2 - is the content of arterial oxygen in 100 ml of arterial blood, measuring the oxygen dissolved in the blood plasma and the oxygen carried by hemoglobin in the red blood cells. Normal is 20 vol% or 20 ml/dl. C_vO_2 is the same measure of mixed venous blood from the pulmonary artery and C_cO_2 is the theoretical amount of oxygen in the pulmonary capillary

Capnograph - a device for measuring carbon dioxide (CO_2)

Cardiac output (Q) - this is the amount of blood the heart pumps in one minute; usually 4 or 5 liters, there are various methods of measuring cardiac output.

Cellular respiration - a number of biochemical reactions and processes that take place in the cells to convert chemical energy from primarily glucose (sugar) by burning in the presence of oxygen molecules converting the energy stored in sugar into adenosine triphosphate (ATP), and then release waste products primarily water and carbon dioxide

Central venous pressure (CVP) - pressure in the large veins (vena cava) returning to the right heart. A very important measurement of circulatory function

Chronic bronchitis - a form of COPD, chronic obstructive pulmonary disease

cmH$_2$O - is a measure of pressure like pounds per square inch (PSI). cmH$_2$O unit is the amount of pressure that is caused by being under a water column one centimeter (about a half inch) high. One cmH_2O is not very much pressure. For example, 1.0 PSI is = 70 cmH_2O

CMV – continuous mechanical ventilation, a generic acronym for any type of mechanical ventilation that is not just intermittent treatments

Compliance - lung and thoracic compliance, is a measure of the lung and chest wall ability to stretch and expand. It is calculated by dividing the tidal volume by the amount of pressure it took to deliver the tidal volume. It is best measured at a point where there is no air flow in order to keep the measurement clean from the pressure required to overcome airway resistance. Normal compliance is $200ml/cmH_2O$

Compliance, static - lung/ thoracic compliance measured at plateau pressure where there is no air movement

Chronic Obstructive Pulmonary Disease (COPD) - is a preventable and treatable disease with some significant extrapulmonary effects that may contribute to the severity in individual patients. Its pulmonary component is characterized by airflow limitation that is not fully reversible. The airflow limitation is usually progressive and associated with an abnormal inflammatory response of the lung to noxious particles or gases. GOLD definition 2006

Control mode - this is ventilator mode of breathing where the ventilator does all the breathing, and the patient cannot trigger or breathe spontaneously. It is seldom used on purpose. By default, it is often the mode of the patient in a medical coma. Since the patient is doing nothing and the ventilator is doing everything it is essentially control mode even though the actual setting might be assist-control or SIMV mode

CO_2 - the chemical equation for carbon dioxide, one carbon atom and two oxygen atoms

CO-Oximeter - a laboratory instrument that measures S_aO_2, $S_{co}O_2$, $S_{met}O_2$, these are respectively alpha hemoglobin oxygen saturation, methemoglobin saturation and carboxy hemoglobin saturation. Alpha hemoglobin is normal hemoglobin, methemoglobin is an abnormal hemoglobin and carboxyhemoglobin is hemoglobin combined with carbon monoxide in carbon monoxide poisoning.

CPAP - continuous positive airway pressure, CPAP is during spontaneous breathing only. Continuous airway pressure during mechanical breaths is called PEEP. If it is a mix of mechanical and spontaneous breaths usually PEEP is the chosen acronym

CPR Code status - is probably best described in Chapter 2, POLST. However, individual hospitals have their own versions. In the simplest form they are "Full Code" or do everything, "No Code" only comfort care, and some partial code in between that describes which invasive procedures, including ventilators, the patient may or may not want

Deadspace ventilation - deadspace ventilation where air breathed into the lung goes to an area without any blood flow and cannot exchange oxygen and carbon dioxide. Anatomic deadspace is normal airways that don't exchange gases like the trachea and bronchi, Alveolar deadspace is abnormal because it should have blood flow and exchange oxygen and carbon dioxide, Mechanical deadspace is any part of the ventilator patient circuit that has both inspired and expired air going back and forth each breath (rebreathed)

Diaphragm muscle - the large, thin, dome shaped, primary muscle of ventilation that separates the chest and abdominal cavities

Direct relationship - type of relationship whereby if there is a change with one variable, then there will be a corresponding change in the other variable. If one goes up the other goes up. For example, there is a direct relationship between pushing on the gas pedal and the speed of the car. Push harder the car goes faster

Dynamic compliance - static lung compliance is the change in volume for any given applied pressure. Dynamic lung compliance is the compliance of the lung at any given time during actual movement of air

Emboli, pulmonary - Pulmonary embolism (PE) is a blockage of an artery in the lungs by a piece of material (blood clot, air bubble, blob of bacteria, lump of fat) that has moved from elsewhere in the body through the bloodstream (embolism)

Endotracheal tube - is a catheter that is inserted through the mouth or nose into the trachea for the primary purpose of establishing and maintaining a patent airway, connecting to a ventilator, and providing a route for airway suctioning. It has a balloon tip in the trachea to create a seal and it is secured to the patient's head with a tube fastening device or adhesive tape

End-tidal carbon dioxide (ETCO$_2$) is measured with a capnograph and is a non-invasive method of approximating the P_aCO_2 or arterial carbon dioxide level

EPAP - Expiratory Positive Airway Pressure is usually a setting on NIV that is the amount of pressure held on the airway during the expiratory phase of spontaneous breathing. It is in a sense like PEEP during invasive mechanical ventilation

Esophagus - the food tube from the throat (pharynx) to the stomach

ETCO$_2$ – end-tidal carbon dioxide, is measured with a capnograph and is a non-invasive method of approximating the PaCO2, or arterial carbon dioxide level

Expiratory time - the length of time the ventilator or patient is in the expiratory phase of the respiratory cycle or breathing out

Expiratory Time Constant (RC$_{exp}$) = **Expiratory Resistance (R$_{exp}$) x Lung Thoracic Compliance (C$_{LT}$).** In words, it is a calculation of how long it will take to empty the lungs by passive exhalation which is not linear

Expiratory Trigger Sensitivity (ETS) – is the criteria that terminates inspiratory phase in spontaneous breathing with pressure support ventilation. It is also called an expiratory flow trigger, 'ESENS', 'End Inspiration', 'Flow Cycle', etc. depending on the brand of ventilator

f – respiratory rate, the number of breaths a patient gets or takes in one minute, normal is 12 - 16/min

F$_I$O$_2$ - fraction of inspired oxygen, the fraction of the inspired air that is oxygen expressed as a decimal fraction like 0.40 is equal to air with 40% oxygen. ICU staff refer to that same oxygen level as "40% oxygen" or "F$_I$O$_2$ is 40". F$_I$O$_2$ is more medically proper. % oxygen is more commonly used

Flow trigger - this is when the ventilator detects a small change in air flow generated by the patient and gives the ventilator patient a breath

Functional Residual Capacity (FRC) - the amount of air left in the lungs at the end of a relaxed exhalation. It can be achieved by just relaxing after any breath.

Hand ventilation - ventilating a patient by squeezing a manual resuscitation bag. Sometimes slangily referred to as "bagging the patient"

Hematocrit - is a blood test that measures how much of a person's blood is made up of red blood cells. This is important because red blood cells carry oxygen from the lungs to the body. Hematocrit (Hct) is normally 36 - 45% of the blood.

Hemoglobin - is an oxygen carrying protein in red blood cells. Hemoglobin gives red blood cells their color when carrying oxygen from the lungs to the rest of the body. With less oxygen hemoglobin turns blue when carrying carbon dioxide back to the lungs to be exhaled

HME - "heat moisture exchanger" is a filter that removes heat and moisture from the patient's exhaled air and places it back into the air of the next breath going into the patient

Hypercapnia/Hypercarbia - elevated carbon dioxide (CO_2) levels in the blood. Carbon dioxide is a product of the body's metabolism and is normally breathed out through the lungs. Caused by increased metabolism or decreased minute volume

Hyperpnea - deeper than normal breaths, greater than normal tidal volume

Hyperventilation - P_aCO_2 less than 35 – 45 mmHg. Does not mean breathing fast (tachypnea) or deeply (hyperpnea); although, that is what happens when normal people breath fast and deeply.

Hypoxemia - low oxygen in the blood, P_aO_2 less than 80 - 100 mmHg, S_pO_2 less than 93 - 99%

Hypoxia - a general term describing less than normal amount of oxygen available to the body tissues

Hypoxic drive - this is a name for breathing stimulated by oxygen receptors located in the aorta and carotid arteries. When oxygen in the blood gets too low, about P_aO_2 = 50 mmHg (normal is 80 - 100 mmHg) or about S_pO_2 = 80% (normal is 95 - 99%) the peripheral chemoreceptors in the carotid and aortic bodies stimulate the brain to breath more. This is breathing driven by hypoxemia. Normal stimulation to breathe comes from central chemoreceptors that monitor pH/P_aCO_2

Hypoventilation - P_aCO_2 greater than 35 - 45 mmHg.

Hypocapnia/Hypocarbia - lowered carbon dioxide (CO_2) levels in the blood. Carbon dioxide is a product of the body's metabolism and is normally breathed out through the lungs. Caused by decreased metabolism or increased minute volume

ICU Delirium - an acute and fluctuating disturbance of consciousness and cognition, is a common manifestation of acute brain dysfunction in critically ill patients, occurring in up to 80% of the sickest intensive care unit (ICU) populations

ICU nurse - a highly trained nurse that can work in the complex ICU environment, CCRN is the National credential for these best of the best nurses

ICU Psychosis - Psychotic episode(s) occurring within 24 hours after entering the intensive care unit in people with no previous history of psychosis; related to sleep deprivation, overstimulation, and time spent on life support systems

Inspiratory hold - this is a maneuver to hold the patient at peak inspiration. Inspiratory flow will be stopped, and exhalation will not be allowed to begin until the end of the inspiratory hold maneuver. This is used to calculate compliance, and it is used in lung recruitment procedures

Inspiratory time - the length of time the ventilator or patient is in the inspiratory phase of the respiratory cycle, or breathing in

IPAP - Inspiratory Positive Airway Pressure is usually a setting on NIV that is the amount of peak inspiratory pressure during spontaneous breathing. It is in a sense like pressure support during invasive mechanical ventilation

Intensivist - is a board-certified physician who provides special care for critically ill patients, the intensivist has advanced training and experience in treating this complex type of patient with multi-system failure. Intensivists typically come from an anesthesiology, pulmonology, or internal medicine background.

Inverse relationship - type of relationship whereby if there is a change with one variable, then there will be an opposite change in the other variable. If one goes up the other goes down. For example, there is an inverse relationship between pushing on the brake pedal and the speed of the car. Push harder the car goes slower

Left Heart - the heart is actually two blood pumps stuck together and work in synchrony. The left side of the heart is most powerful and pumps blood to the whole body. The right heart pumps blood to the lungs and back to the left heart

Liter - a metric measure of fluids, one liter is about one quart. (1.0 liters = 1.06 quarts)

Manual resuscitator - is a portable, handheld device that self inflates that can be used to ventilate people by applying a mask to the face and squeezing the bag, "in goes the good air." it has a two-way valve to allow the person to exhale before the bag is squeezed again. For patients with tracheal tubes the face mask is replaced with an adapter to the tracheal tube

MAP - mean airway pressure, this is the average airway pressure over a period of time or number of breaths, as MAP increases P_aO_2 is likely to increase. The direct way of increasing MAP is to increase the PEEP

Mechanical deadspace - is any part of the ventilator patient circuit that has both inspired and expired air going back and forth each breath (rebreathed)

Medical coma - sedation and analgesia in order to tolerate the endotracheal tube, to lie down in the same position for a long time, to prevent dysynchrony with the ventilator, to tolerate many of the procedures, for optimization of oxygenation and for patient safety

Metabolism, body - is the process by which your body breaks down what you eat and drink and converts it into energy. During this biochemical process, calories in food and beverages are combined with oxygen to release the energy our body needs to function

Minute volume - the volume of air a person breathes in one minute expressed in liters/minute

Mode – modes of ventilation include spontaneous, SIMV, and assist-control, and many other acronyms and proprietary terms

Near Drowning - is a term for those who survive the struggle against drowning

Near Fatal Asthma - asthma so serious that it results in intubation and placing on a ventilator

NIV - non-invasive ventilation is mechanical ventilation connected to the patient with a face mask rather than a tracheal tube. It is commonly called BiPAP which is a proprietary term

OVP - "operational verification procedure" is a standardized, documented testing procedure for a ventilator that has been cleaned and set up for the next patient. OVP ensures the ventilator functions and alarms are all working well

Oxygen toxicity - exposure of the lungs to greater than 60% oxygen for periods exceeding 24-48 hours can lead to severe, irreversible pulmonary fibrosis

Oxygenation failure - respiratory failure characterized by inability to get enough oxygen into the lungs and then getting the oxygen into the bloodstream

P0.1 – airway occlusion pressure, this is a pressure measured in the first 0.1 seconds of inspiration, or rather first 100 millisecs of inspiration. It is measured by an embedded ventilator computer. P0.1 during normal breathing is 1 - 2 cmH_2O. If it is greater than 3 - 5 cmH_2O probably the patient will fail a spontaneous breathing trial (SBT)

P_aCO_2 - partial pressure of carbon dioxide in the arterial blood. This is the most commonly measure of how well ventilation is matching metabolism in the body. The blood sample for this test must be taken from an artery, which is a pulsating blood vessel, not a vein

P_aO_2 - partial pressure of oxygen in the arterial blood. This is the most common measure of oxygen in the body. The blood sample for this test must be taken from an artery, which is a pulsating blood vessel, not a vein

PCIRV - pressure control ventilation with inverse I:E ratio, this is just PCV with the inspiratory time longer than expiratory time used to increase oxygenation by increasing MAP

PCV – pressure-controlled ventilation, a mode of ventilation where the peak pressure is set rather than tidal volume. In PCV the amount of tidal volume varies with the patient's resistance and compliance. PCV can be AC-PCV or SIMV-PCV

Peak inspiratory pressure (PIP) - is measured when the full tidal volume is in the patient's lungs. PIP is the highest pressure reached during inspiration

P_ECO_2 = 35 – 43 mmHg., where P is partial pressure, E is end-tidal and CO_2 is carbon dioxide. A non-invasive way to monitor/estimate carbon dioxide in the blood

PEEP - Positive End-Expiratory Pressure is during mechanical breaths only. If it is a mix of mechanical and spontaneous breaths usually PEEP is chosen over the acronym CPAP. PEEP holds air in the lungs at the end of expiration and increases FRC which in turn may increase the P_aO_2

Permissive hypercapnia - is allowing the ventilator patient to have an abnormally high P_aCO_2 and is evoked whenever the healthcare team fails to be able adequately ventilate the patient within "acceptable" limits

Pneumonia - a bacterial, viral, fungal or other infection of the lungs. It is a serious and sometimes fatal disease

Pneumothorax - the presence of air or gas in the cavity between the lungs and the chest wall, causing collapse of the lung. This is caused by a hole in the lung letting air leak into the space just outside the lung, but inside the chest wall.

POLST (Physician Orders for Life-Sustaining Treatment) is an abbreviated type of Advanced Directive that states directly "Do or Do not Resuscitate" if the patient has no pulse or is not breathing. It can further specify if the person has a pulse and breathing that they may only want certain medical options or procedures.

P_{ramp}, **(rise time)** – the set amount of time the ventilator is allowed from the beginning of inspiration to reach PSV and/ or PCV pressure level. Rise time is how fast the ventilator accelerates the flowrate to reach some higher-pressure goal

Pressure trigger - this is when the ventilator detects a small drop in airway pressure and gives the ventilator patient a breath

PSV – pressure support ventilation is an adjunct to spontaneous breathing where the ventilator gives a positive pressure boost to the patient's spontaneous breath

PS-ILI - is generated by intense inspiratory effort yielding: (A) swings in transpulmonary pressure (i.e. lung stress); (B) abnormal increases in transvascular pressure, producing pulmonary edema; (C) an intra-lung shift of air between different lung zones; (D) diaphragmatic injury

Pulmonary artery - the main artery from the right heart to the lungs, it carries "unoxygenated" blood from all over the body, mixed together, to the lungs to get rid of carbon dioxide and pick up oxygen

Pulmonary artery pressure (PAP) - the blood pressure in the main pulmonary artery, normally 24/10 mmHg. It is a much lower pressure system because it only has to pump the blood a short distance to the lungs

Pulmonary artery occlusion pressure (PAOP) - the pulmonary artery catheter has a small balloon tip. If the catheter is properly placed in a smaller branch of the pulmonary artery, the balloon can be inflated and seal off the artery. When this happens, the remaining pressure is the pressure through the lungs being pushed back by the left atrium. This allows the ICU team to get information on left heart back pressure. Normal 6 -12 mmHg

Pulmonary artery (Swan-Ganz) catheter - is a long diagnostic catheter introduced through a larger vein, pushed toward the right heart and floated through the heart into the pulmonary artery until the balloon "wedges", blocking the blood flow in that pulmonary artery. The balloon is then deflated to allow blood flow. A PA catheter can measure central venous pressure in the right atrium through one port, PAP and PAOP and oxygen saturation through the distal port and a sensing wire probe built into the catheter

Pulmonary capillary - are the tiny, microscopic, blood vessels between the pulmonary arteries and the pulmonary veins. The wall of the pulmonary capillary is up against the wall of the alveolus so oxygen and carbon dioxide can diffuse in and out of the blood to the lungs.

Pulmonary edema - a condition caused by excess fluid in the lungs. This fluid collects in the numerous air sacs in the lungs. Left heart problems often cause pulmonary edema. A small amount of pulmonary edema sounds like Rice Krispies through a stethoscope. A large amount of pulmonary edema fulminates out of the mouth, nose, or tracheal tube in a pink froth

Pulmonary emphysema - "a common, preventable, and treatable disease that is characterized by persistent respiratory symptoms and airflow limitation that is due to airway and/or alveolar abnormalities usually caused by significant exposure to noxious particles or gases." GOLD Guidelines

Pneumatic - operated by air or gas under pressure, like a pneumatic hammer or jackhammer

Pneumothorax - air outside the lungs but inside the chest wall that is most often caused by a hole in the lung and air leaking out into the pleural space.

Pneumothorax, tension - This is when the pneumothorax is large, collapses the lung and begins to increase pressure in the collapsed side of the chest. This pressure can push the heart and the other lung into collapse and may result in sudden death if not identified and resolved immediately.

Q_s/Q_T - the classic equation for calculating right-to left intrapulmonary shunt. It requires an arterial blood sample and data from a pulmonary artery catheter. Q = cardiac output, S = amount of R-L intrapulmonary shunt, and T = the total blood flow to the lungs

Resistance, airway - frictional forces opposing the flow of air; the length of the airway and size of the airway are important factors for airway resistance which is measured in centimeters of water/liter of air/second, or how much pressure it takes to blow air through a tube of a certain length and diameter

Right heart - the heart is actually two blood pumps stuck together and work in synchrony. The right side of the heart pumps blood to the lungs and back to the left heart. The left heart is most powerful and pumps blood to the whole body and back to the right heart

Rise time (P_{ramp}) – or pressure ramp, is the set amount of time the ventilator is allowed from the beginning of inspiration to reach PSV and/or PCV pressure level. Rise time is how fast the ventilator accelerates the flowrate to reach some pressure goal

RSB or RSBI – rapid shallow breathing index is the ratio of respiratory frequency to tidal volume (f/VT). As an example, a patient who has a respiratory rate of 25 breaths/min and a tidal volume of 250 mL/breath has an RSBI of (25 breaths/min)/ (.25 L) = 100 breaths/min/L. Generally, an RSBI < 105 predicts a patient will succeed in a spontaneous breathing trial (SBT)

S_aO_2 - arterial oxygen saturation, measured with CO-oximeter or calculated, normal S_aO_2 = 95 - 97%

SBT - spontaneous breathing trial is done each morning to see if the ventilator patient can breathe on their own. SBT is currently the best indicator if the patient can be taken off the ventilator when their underlying problem has been resolved

Sensitivity - is the relative ease with which the patient can signal the ventilator to get a breath on demand. Sensitivity is sometimes called "trigger sensitivity" or "trigger"

Shunt, Right-to-Left Intrapulmonary - shunted blood refers to blood that bypasses where it is supposed to go. In this case the blood is supposed to go from the right side of the heart to the lung and pick up oxygen; instead, it goes to lung tissue that is collapsed, filled with fluid or otherwise not ventilated. This shunted blood returns to the left heart and then to the rest of the body short of oxygen

Sigh – periodic hyperinflation of the lungs.

SIMV – synchronized intermittent mandatory ventilation, this is a mode of ventilation where the patient can breathe spontaneously while the ventilator will give them synchronized machine breaths at a certain rate per minute. For example, with an SIMV of 6 the patient may be breathing 15 times per minute; the ventilator will wait until the patient is ready to take one of these breaths and give them a machine breath 6 times per minute. This allows the patient to take deep breaths, sigh and be more comfortable while at a lower MAP than assist-control or control mode ventilation

S_pO_2 - Oxygen saturation measured by a non-invasive (finger sensor) pulse oximeter, under normal conditions S_pO_2 is close to S_aO_2 and P_aO_2, so it is a great way to monitor the patient's oxygen and therefore effectiveness of breathing.

Spontaneous Breathing Trial (SBT) - SBT is the ICU staff giving ventilator patients a chance to breathe on their own each morning. This is done after most sedation wears off. If the patient can successfully breathe for 30 mins to 2 hours, it may be time to get rid of the ventilator.

Spontaneous Mode – spontaneous ventilation; breaths initiated and defined by the patient. Normal ventilation is spontaneous ventilation. On a ventilator spontaneous ventilation may include CPAP, PS, and other ventilator adjustments to suit the patient like rise time and expiratory trigger sensitivity

Spontaneous ventilation - breaths initiated and defined by the patient. Normal ventilation is spontaneous ventilation. On a ventilator spontaneous ventilation may include CPAP, PS, and other ventilator adjustments to suit the patient like rise time and expiratory trigger sensitivity

S_vO_2 - mixed venous oxygen saturation measured by an oximetric sensor floating deep inside the pulmonary artery or from a blood sample taken from a pulmonary artery catheter. Under normal conditions S_vO_2 is close to 75%, so it is a great way to monitor how much oxygen the patient's body is extracting from the hemoglobin from all over the body. Good to help assess the efficiency of breathing

Tachypnea - abnormally rapid breathing, usually more than 20 breaths per minute

Thoracic cavity - is the inside of the chest, the cavity containing the heart, lungs, great blood vessels. The esophagus runs down through the thoracic cavity. The thoracic cavity is an inverted cone shape and bounded by the rib cage and diaphragm

Tidal volume - is the volume of air in milliliters (1000 ml = about a quart) of a single normal breath. Tidal volume times breaths per minute = minute volume

Trachea - commonly known as the (windpipe), the large airway connecting the bottom of the larynx (voice box) to where it divides into two mainstem bronchi that go into the right and left lung. The trachea is a rigid structure with cartilaginous, C-shaped rings about 3 - 5 inches in length

Tracheostomy - is a hole that surgeons make through the front of the neck and into the windpipe (trachea)

Tracheostomy tube - is inserted through the hole (tracheostomy) and secured with a strap around the neck. Its purpose is to keep the airway open for breathing. With ventilators the tracheostomy tube will have a balloon located on the end in the trachea to create a seal for positive pressure ventilation and a ventilator adapter on the outside end.

Transpulmonary pressure - (P$_l$) has traditionally been used to describe the pressure difference (or pressure drop) across the whole lung, including the airways and lung tissue, and is defined as the pressure at the airway opening (Pao) minus the pressure in the pleural space (Ppl), Pl = Pao – Ppl. In other words, it is normally the difference in the air pressure in one's open mouth and the pressure generated by the respiratory muscles to suck in a breath.

Trigger - see sensitivity

VCV – volume-controlled ventilation, a mode of ventilation where the tidal volume is set rather than peak airway pressure. In VCV the peak airway pressure varies with the patient's resistance and compliance. VCV can be AC-VCV or SIMV-VCV

V_D/V_T - deadspace volume to tidal volume ratio. V_D is the amount of wasted ventilation or deadspace ventilation where air breathed into the lung goes to an area without any blood flow and cannot exchange oxygen and carbon dioxide. V_T is another abbreviation of tidal volume. So, this is how much of a patient's tidal volume is being wasted. Normally about 15 - 30% is considered wasted because it just goes in and out of the tracheal and bronchi.

Veins - are blood vessels that bring back blood that has been used by the body to the heart to get pumped to the lungs and refreshed. Most blood test samples are taken from veins

Ventilatory failure - inability to breathe enough to keep carbon dioxide at normal levels in the blood, failure to ventilate, hypoventilation

VILI - ventilator-induced lung injury (VILI) can result in pulmonary edema, barotrauma, volutrauma, and worsening hypoxemia that can prolong mechanical ventilation, lead to multi-system organ dysfunction, and increased mortality.

Vital Capacity - is the deepest breath we can take in or blow out, it is typically measure by asking someone to breathe in as deeply as possible and blast it all the way out with a maximum effort.

Volutrauma - lung injury caused by alveolar overdistension, overinflation

ACKNOWLEDGEMENTS

Many thanks to my wife, Yoko Shimoyoshi, for her editing, encouragement, and ideas for the book. Thanks to Gavin Lamb and Kimiyo Yamasaki for editing and their ideas. Many thanks to Amy Sanderson and Philip Couturier for invaluable advice, beautiful graph generation, formatting, and publishing. Thanks to Rani Sanderson for marketing and distribution ideas. Thanks to Darlene Mauro for encouragement and help with the title. I appreciate the members of my book club, Book Club Hawaii, and the Society for Mechanical Ventilation for their on-going encouragement.

CPSIA information can be obtained
at www.ICGtesting.com
Printed in the USA
FSHW021148060421
80134FS